Find out how easy it is to save yourself and our world!

Here's what some of our best and unbiased minds and non-political and non-profit organizations say:

"Nothing will benefit human health and increase the chances for survival of life on earth as much as the evolution of a vegetarian diet."
- *Albert Einstein*

"A low-fat plant-based diet would not only lower the heart attack rate about 85%, but would lower the cancer rate 60%."
- *William Castelli, M.D., Director, Framingham Health Study; National Heart, Lung & Blood Institute*

"Healthy Eating Costs Less: Contrary to popular belief, a recent study published in the Journal of the American Diabetic Association finds that healthy eating can reduce a family's overall food costs. The study states that high fat, low nutrition foods often cost more than fruits and vegetables." Eating healthy can save the average family more than 25% of their annual food costs, plus the added benefit of being happier, more productive and having big savings on health care costs.
- *MSNBC (9/13/02)*

"Global warming has emerged as the most serious environmental threat of the 21st century... Only by taking action now can we insure that future generations will not be put at risk."
- *Letter to the president from 49 Nobel Prize-winning scientists*

"We would save more water by not eating a pound of beef than we would by not showering for one year."
- *University of California Agricultural Extension Soil and Water Specialists*

"The amount of water that goes into a 1,000 pound steer would float a Naval destroyer."
- *Newsweek, Feb. 22, 1981*

"The production of every quarter-pound hamburger in the U.S. causes the loss of five times the burger's weight in topsoil."
- *Stuff: The Secret Lives of Everyday Things (Seattle: Northwest Environment Watch, 1997). John Ryan & Alan Durning*

"Dairies are the single largest source of water pollution... Our volunteers frequently encounter massive discharges of dairy waste that literally cauterize waterways and kill fish..."
- *Deltakeeper, an environmental group that monitors California's waterways*

"The number of Californians whose drinking water is threatened by contamination from dairy manure: 20 million (65% of state population)."
- *"State Dairy Farmers try to clean up their act", Clone*

"A cultural shift toward a plant-based diet would be a substantial step toward saving our remaining rainforests. It takes far less agricultural land to produce a plant-based diet than to produce meat...Since forests absorb carbon dioxide and produce oxygen, the movement toward a plant-based diet would provide our children with more plentiful oxygen to breathe, an atmosphere with fewer greenhouse gases, and a more stable climate."
- *The Food Revolution, John Robbins*

"In a world where an estimated one in every six people goes hungry every day, the politics of meat consumption are increasingly heated, since meat production is an inefficient use of grain - the grain is used more efficiently when consumed directly by humans. Continued growth of meat output is dependent on feeding grains to animals, creating competition for grain between affluent meat eaters and the world's poor."
- Worldwatch Institute

"Meat contributes an extraordinary significant percentage of saturated fat in the American diet."
- Marion Nestle, Chair of the Nutrition Dept., New York University

"Studies indicate that vegetarians often have lower morbidity and mortality rates...Not only is mortality from coronary artery disease lower in vegetarians than non-vegetarians, but vegetarian diets have also been successful in arresting coronary artery disease. Scientific data suggest positive relationships between a vegetarian diet and reduced risk for...obesity, coronary artery disease, hypertension, diabetes, and some types of cancer."
- American Dietetic Association

"The beef industry has contributed to more deaths than all the wars of this century, all natural disasters, and all automobile accidents combined. If beef is your idea of 'real food for real people', you'd better live real close to a real good hospital."
- Neal Barnard, M.D., President, Physicians Committee for Responsible Medicine

"A report by the USDA estimates that 89% of U.S. beef ground into patties contains traces of deadly E.coli strain."
- Reuters News Service, August 10, 2000

Diets low in saturated fat and cholesterol that include 20-25g of ANUTRA® a day may reduce the risk of heart disease.

Eating more vegetables, fruits and ANUTRA® may be as effective at reducing cholesterol as medication.

Also consider these important facts:

- 30 million Americans are food insecure.

- Nearly 800 million people around the world are hungry and approximately 200 million of them are children under 5 years of age.

- 31% of adults in the U.S. are obese - up from 23% a decade ago. More than 60% of Americans are overweight.

- 1 in 3 Americans born after 2000 will develop Type II diabetes, 1 in 100 are now born with autism, 1 in 8 US births is premature with many birth defects and deaths.

- Among children over 5 years, 30% are either seriously overweight or at risk of becoming seriously overweight. 21% of 2 to 5 year old children are overweight or at risk of being overweight.

- Approximately 70% of the world's population are lactose intolerant.

- There are 17 million people in the United States who have diabetes. Type 2 diabetes accounts for 90% to 95% of diabetes. Type 2 diabetes is nearing epidemic proportions, due to an increased number of older Americans, and a greater prevalence of obesity and sedentary lifestyles, especially among children. (ADA)

- Water used to produce 1 pound of U.S. beef: 2,500 gallons. Water used to produce 1 pound of grain: 60 gallons.

- The amount of grain needed to produce 1 pound of U.S. beef is almost 17 pounds. (USDA)

- More than 90% of all the grain produced in the U.S. is used to feed livestock.

- Livestock account for 12% to 20% of overall global methane emissions.

- Percentage of eight-year old child's daily value for saturated fat in one Double Whopper with cheese: more than 200%!

- Amount spent annually by the dairy industry on the "milk mustache" ads: $190 million

- Amount spent annually by the National Cancer Society promoting fruits and vegetables: only $1 million

- Annual U.S. medical costs directly attributable to meat consumption: $60 - $120 BILLION

- Antibiotics allowed in U.S. cow's milk: 80

- After WWII, the U.S. was ranked first in the world in life expectancy. Today, we are ranked a dismal 44th.

Photo Credits: Robert Wiley, Wiley Foto

Editors: Angelo S. Morini; Brian J. Morini, GS Doctor of Pharmacy;
Dr. Wayne Coates; Dr. Debbrah Harding,M.D.;
Douglas A. Walsh, M.D., D.O.; Dr. William J. Robbins, M.D.
;

Technical Editor: Gilbran Laureano

Recipe Technical Advisor: Victoria Prada Arribas

Cover & Book Design: Jamie L. Morini

Manufactured in the United States of America
Published March 15, 2008
1st Edition Printing, March 2008

ISBN: 978-0-981669-0-7

Nature's "Best Kept Secret"

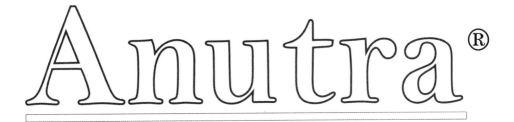

Anutra®

&

World's Healthiest Whole Food

**ELIMINATE OVER 150,000
CALORIES ANNUALLY
THAT IS 35 OR MORE POUNDS!**

by
Angelo S. Morini

Table of Contents

Introduction

I got my introduction to the health food business back in the late 1960's, I literally experimented in my father's butcher shop trying to invent a different way to make cheese. I was in the pizza business and thought it would be a great way to save money on cheese costs. I probably was half-mad at the time. I was not a scientist or a chemist, but I was a young and ambitious person who was determined to figure it out, and, I did.

When a Framingham Study in 1972 first told us of the dangers of cholesterol in our foods and its relation to coronary heart disease, I began to think. Wouldn't it be great to remove the bad elements of cheese so it was not harmful to us? I went back to my father's butcher shop for more experimenting. This time it took me a bit longer, but I got it. My claim to fame is that I initiated the cholesterol, low-fat, trans-fatty acids, and lactose free movement in the United States and was the first person in the world to market a dairy alternative with these attributes. That was in 1972, and it was a time when very few people were interested.

Well, as the saying goes, we've come a long way since then. Today, my new company, ValuHealth, distributes a new cultivar of an amazingly exciting grain.

I became interested in *Salvia Hispanica L.* (ANUTRA®) after receiving a call from Nobel Prize Winning associates, introducing me to the grain. I received samples and began consuming the product on a regular basis and to my amazement, old nagging health problems disappeared. I had a life long problem with psoriasis, peptic ulcer and being an avid exerciser, my muscles were always sore. All of these problems simply disappeared and I became really interested and began a major scientific investigation that resulted in amazement and ANUTRA® becoming the World's Healthiest Whole Food.

ANUTRA® is a new leader in what is the fastest growing segment in the food industry today - the healthy, natural, and organic foods category. There are multiple drivers behind this major category growth, including demographic and societal changes, consumer perception, favorable regulation, and wider mass market availability. The most important societal change affecting the category growth is that today's informed consumers are becoming more aware of the reasons we should consume more protein from plant-based foods. These reasons include our health and nutrition, our environment, and economics (including world hunger). These are the driving forces behind my writing this book.

With increasing media attention providing consumers with the awareness of the negative effects of growth hormones and antibiotics injected in our livestock; pollution of our rivers and streams from slaughterhouses and feedlots; the effects of greenhouse gases on our climate; the pollution caused by methane emissions (from livestock); the health dangers of eating foods with saturated fat, cholesterol, harmful preservatives, and artificial ingredients; and many other important factors, the realization that we must increase our intake of plant proteins is becoming more widely known.

In addition, the alarming rising levels of obesity (especially in children), diabetes, cardiovascular disease, and cancer are of great medical concern. Prevention needs to become increasingly more important to us; we need to make better food choices and lead more active lifestyles to try to take control of our own health.

When I was growing up, polio affected 1 in 3000. Today, autism affects 1 in 100 children born and is rising worldwide. Also, 1 in 8 births is premature and many of these babies do not make it or are severely handicapped for life. We are what we eat and we must get smarter and know what is good for us to prevent these tragedies.

In my new book about ANUTRA®, I recommend simple eating and lifestyle changes which will affect how we feel, how we look, how we act, the quality of the air we breathe, the land we love, the water we drink, our climate, and the more than 800 million people around the world who are hungry. How civilized is our world if we allow one million children to die needlessly each week? I will tell you how simple it is to dramatically reduce your caloric intake and improve your health by changing very little in your lifestyle and, at the same time, help the world economy, the environment, and ultimately our fellow man.

So, please give it a try - ANUTRASIZE™ I'm telling you, you won't believe the difference it can make in how you feel and how easy it will be to maintain your proper weight. And, you will also know you are helping others at the same time. ANUTRASIZE™ is an important and healthy life-change that is so simple yet so physically beneficial and spiritually uplifting. Thank you for this opportunity to tell you more. If this knowledge and approach to healthy living helps you improve your life, I encourage you to pass it along and share these principles with others you love and care about.

Angelo S. Morini

OUR PRECIOUS CHILDREN

Nothing makes me more sad than what has happened to our children in our beloved U.S.A.. I, and many others, have been telling the shakers and so called movers "the inteligencia" for years about the consequences of a bad diet like the ones we Americans are on. For the first time in our history, our children will not live as long as their parents. We are ranked 44th in life expectancy down from number #1 shortly after World War II. This is a national tragedy that must be stopped now! No one wants this to continue but unless we change some things, everything will just get worse. Here is how bad it is now. One in 3 born after the year 2000 will be diabetic. One in 8 births in the United States of America is premature causing many deaths and birth defects. One in 100 births is autistic, Eighteen percent of our children are obese and growing at an alarming rate that will deteriorate their health in the short and long term. And the list of maladies and terrible consequences goes on and on. How can we change all this for the better? Here are my suggestions:

The farm subsidy program started by president Roosevelt in 1938 to prepare the UNITED STATES for World War II was put in place to last only until we were victorious. Well, the program has grown to approximately $300 billion in 2007, but no relief in sight. The proponents of the farm-bill say that without government subsidies, Americans will starve. The free market system has made the USA the best country in the world in so many ways, we do not need this type of control because it affects the very core health of our children and everyone else. Here is how it works:

The USA government supports meat and dairy producers and the food for these animals. An astounding 90% of all grain grown in America goes to feed animal and is subsidized (not much fruit or vegetables are subsidized). These subsidized meat and dairy products find their way to our schools because of the schools wanting to save tax-payers money. This almost free food is gladly served to our children, lots of meat and dairy products loaded with harmful fats, lots of salt, sugar and a bunch of harmful chemicals that do not have to be listed in ingredients due to big pharmaceutical and commodity food producers' influence.

These fats that are subsized both plant and animal are disastrous to our children in two big ways: 1. they are high in cholesterol, saturated fats and the omega-3's, omega-6's are out of sync. The correct ratio being 3:1 omega-3's to omega-6's. The average ratio for our children is 20:1 omega-6's to omega-3's. This is very unhealthy for proper cell development and causes our children to be much less than they cold be if fed a proper diet. 2. When you feed a child at a very young age high fats, salty and sweet foods, you program their brains in such a way that they cannot be completely satisfied unless they get their unhealthy foods. They become hooked on these food qualities and they continue these unhealthy habits into adulthood. And, here we are today with this tremendous moral injustice caused by non-other than ourselves. Other powerful interest like the insurance companies, drug companies and some factions of healthcare love it just the way it is because they make more money if we are sick. Knowledge is power and now is the time to get involved with the grassroot levels of your schools and politically at all levels. We can change this if we have the will and I know we all want the best for our children and our Country.

Serving our children ANUTRA® will greatly enhance their overall development and well-being. Children with diabetes, cancer, heart problems and other serious maladies can be helped by consuming ANUTRA®.

ABOUT ANUTRA®

ANUTRA® Nature's Healthiest Whole Food

I believe God created man, heaven, earth, and ANUTRA®. In 1972, I initiated the cholesterol, low-fat, trans-fat and lactose free movement in the United States and the world by introducing the world's number one brand of dairy alternatives. I have also been a student of grains and healthy eating my entire life and have never seen anything that compares to this rediscovery of the world's healthiest whole food. ANUTRA® grain grows from the earth, is dried in the field by the sun, is carefully harvested, is meticulously cleaned, and is quality assured through intense microbiological procedures to ensure that it is perfect for human consumption. ANUTRA® contains very high biologically available protein with all essential amino acids, and its protein level is higher than rice, wheat, corn, oats, soy, and any other plant food. ANUTRA® is also higher in protein than eggs, chicken, turkey, beef, pork, and fish. ANUTRA's® overall nutritional profile is far superior to any other whole food-plant or animal. The omega-3 fatty acids found in ANUTRA® are the perfect ratio and the antioxidants are one of the highest in oxygen radical absorption capacity (ORAC). ANUTRA® contains very high levels of many types of phytonutrients, one in particular being lignans. Sixty-five percent of all anti-cancer drugs utilize lignans in their formulations. ANUTRA® contains six time the amount of calcium as compared to cow's milk and eighty-five percent of the calcium found in the grain is digested and used by the body, as opposed to only thirty-five percent for cow's milk. The calcium found in ANUTRA® is an astonishing fifteen times more than that of cow's milk. Other vitamins, minerals, and nutrients in the grain help make ANUTRA® a nutritional powerhouse. When you include the wonderful digestive properties of ANUTRA® along with its ability to decrease blood pressure, inflammation (CRP levels), glycemic index, clotting (blood-thinning effect comparable to aspirin); the risk of heart disease, cancers, diabetes, osteoporosis, and other serious, chronic diseases, it's no wonder medical and nutritional experts throughout the world are now recognizing ANUTRA® to be "nature's healthiest whole food". ANUTRA® is grown by ANUTRA® FARMS, ensuring consumers that all parameters are diligently maintained. ANUTRA® is the highest biologically available *Salvia Hispanica L.* in the world.

MULTICOLORED ANUTRA® BETTER THAN PLAIN WHITE *SALVIA HISPANICA L.*

Our new multi-colored cultivar of *Salvia Hispanica L.* "ANUTRA®", the world's best, is cultivated utilizing all of God's natural gifts. Some are saying that the segregated all white *Salvia Hispanica L.* grain is superior to our multicolored ANUTRA®. This is totally untrue. Just like other nutritious multi-colored grains including natural brown rice and the rich natural pigmentation of brilliantly colored fruits and vegetables like blueberries, cranberries, peppers and carrots to name a few, lies the magical phytonutrients that contain untold health wonders presently being studies by many scientific clinical researchers including Anutra® Farms. Anutra® Farms has the largest and most qualified staff led by renowned researcher and agricultural scientist, Dr. Wayne Coates, co-author of the book "CHIA" published by the University of Arizona, to assure the efficacy of

ANUTRA® and continue to make the grain the best it can be. Research has shown that black, white, brown, tan and yellow multi-colored ANUTRA® has many different phytonutrients not found in just one color like the plain white grain. The claim that the white grain is superior to the multicolored ANUTRA® is just plain false, period! In contrast, the multicolored grain ANUTRA® having the best overall nutrition and more phytonutrients and flavanoids makes ANUTRA® the healthiest whole food, plant or animal.

THE ULTIMATE RAW FOOD

"Magic potion No. 9" etc., and that is how it is and has been for a long time in the processed food business. Did you know that thousands of ingredients are allowed in our foods without being declared on ingredient statements? Food processor and their lobbyists create their own kingdoms and circumvent the rights of the consumers to know what is in their foods. This is done to enhance their profit positions at the consumers peril. "We are what we eat" and America was a lot better off in every way when the consumer had a clear knowledge about what was in their food.

Preservatives, emulsifiers, artificial flavors, food extenders, unhealthy fats, cholesterol, hidden sodium, lactose and many other ingredients are used in foods that can be very harmful to our health. When we all sat down at the dinner table and ate nutritious home cooked meals, we were all much healthier. America was number one in life span and quality of life after Worlds War II and shortly after that we began our slide into mostly unhealthy processed foods. That changed so many things for the worse like omega-3's going from a healthy ratio (3:1) over omega-6 to an unhealthy percent day average of (20:1) omega-6's to omega-3's not to mention too much cholesterol, saturated fat, and you can imagine the rest.

ANUTRA® is the world's most perfect raw food. It is grown without pesticides, is cured in the fields naturally by the sun, meticulously cleaned and micro-biologically checked to assure you the world's best and healthiest raw food. Use some of the recipes in this book to get you and your family back to the dinner table for so many good reasons.

ANUTRA® NATURE'S HEALTHIEST WHOLE FOOD, is my third book telling the world about world hunger, social injustice, global warming, obesity, dangerous toxins in our food supply, clean air and water, health care cost, and of course healthier eating.

I clearly remember not too many caring about these serious topics years ago when I wrote my first and second book. Just like our present energy crisis that is enslaving us all, our nation is also very sick. When you know that one in a hundred U.S. children are born with autism, one in three born after the year 2000 will get diabetes, 1 in 8 births are premature with many births defects and deaths, health insurance costs and it's social validity being out of control, 17% or more of our Gross National Product is going to health Care that is the highest in the world.

How are we to compete with other nations when their cost is much lower not to mention the serious consequences of the weakening of our very moral fiber.

I remember when the United States was number one in longevity and just about everything else including morality shortly after World War II. Today, we are ranked a dismal and very sad 44th in life expectancy compared to the rest of the world and the obesity crisis and all that goes with it is ripping the heart out of America. I also remember telling the world about these major issues many years ago and nothing was done about it, here we are being enslaved because of our dependence on foreign oil and enormous health-care cost; we cannot afford to wait another 30 years for our health crisis wake-up call like we did with oil. The leaders of our time must have the courage and moral fortitude to do the right things now!

America is truly the greatest country on earth built by great people, but we all know the huge challenges of our times and now is the moment to re-invigorate what we are all about and take the necessary steps that will lead the world to a safer and healthier place. GOD BLESS AMERICA!

THE HEALTHY BENEFITS OF ANUTRA®

Nutritional Benefits

Highest and Safest Source of Omega-3s

Antioxidants, Fiber

& Lignans

*HIGH QUALITY VEGETABLE PROTEIN

*ALL ESSENTIAL AMINO ACIDS

*RICH NATURAL SOURCE OF ANTIOXIDANTS (more than flax or cultivated blueberries)

*ANUTRA® ORAC (Oxygen Radical Absorption Capacity) HYDRO (Umole TE/g) VALUE OF 75 PER GRAM (1,125 per serving)

*5g FIBER PER SERVING

*THIAMIN, SELENIUM, MANGANESE & COPPER

*0g TRANS FAT PER SERVING

*0mg CHOLESTEROL PER SERVING

*NON-GMO, GLUTEN FREE, 100% NATURAL

THE ORIGIN OF A SUPER GRAIN

The non-GMO pesticide free grown super grain ANUTRA® is an exciting new cultivar of an ancient Aztec crop called " Chia" (*Salvia Hispanica L.*).

The incredibly advanced Aztec dynasty, renowned for their outstanding accomplishments in agriculture, horticulture and healing, forged a mighty empire that was able to provide food for over 1 million people. One of the cornerstones of their nutritional foundation was *Salvia Hispanica L.*

The Aztecs used *Salvia Hispanica L.* to attain high energy and endurance. It sustained them on long and arduous hunting and trading expeditions and in battle. Although the grain was vitally important then, its cultivation decreased following the discovery of America. The good news for us is that modern science has rediscovered why this ancient civilization considered this grain so important and significant advancements have been made to make this super grain even better.

ValuHealth is proud to bring you ANUTRA®- a vastly important , novel and nutritious food with tremendous nutritional and health-promoting value. Based on clinical studies conducted on the healthy properties of ANUTRA®, this super grain may soon become one of the first functional foods recommended for maintaining healthy blood sugar and cholesterol levels*

At ValuHealth, we believe that consumers, health professionals and dieticians will realize the importance of including ANUTRA® in our daily diet both by itself and as a vital ingredient in many traditional and specialty foods enjoyed today.

ABOUT VALUHEALTH

The founder and leader of ValuHealth is Angelo S. Morini who is widely known as a pioneer in the health food industry. In 1972, he invented a new, healthier and better way to make dairy products, and was first in US to market a cholesterol free, low fat, trans fat and lactose free product.

Mr. Morini is also the founder and Chairman Emeritus of Galaxy Nutritional Foods the company that has marketed these healthy dairy products for more than 25 years. He revolutionized this important product category with Veggie Brand Dairy Alternatives, the world's number one selling dairy alternative product line made form Veggie Milk (soy, rice and oats). He also introduced the world's largest line of vegan dairy alternatives and rice-based dairy alternatives which together with Veggie brand products, makes Galaxy Nutritional Foods the undisputed leader in the healthy dairy product category around the world.

In continuing his pioneering spirit, Mr. Morini now brings you ANU-TRA® that , he states, "with its superior nutrition and many health-promoting benefits is to date the single most important food discovery ever. You will be amazed at how great you will feel and how you will improve your health, energy and general wellness. I believe that ANUTRA® will become an important staple in our daily diet as more and more of us discover the health promoting properties of this super grain".

Mr. Morini has made many television guest appearances and has lectured throughout the world. His latest book on ANUTRA® explains the ancient Aztec grain and ways to improve your diet and lifestyle through adding ANUTRA® grain either whole or ground into your recipes and eating more plant protein and less animal protein, which will positively affect your health and our world.

ANUTRA® BETTER THAN FLAX

Recent research has identified lignans as key nutrients for maintaining optimal health. Only 2 tablespoons of ANUTRA® provides 1,275 mg of Lignans. Flax contains approximately 50 mg of Lignans for the same serving size.

The amino acid protein profile of ANUTRA® yields a 91% protein quality for ANUTRA® versus a 60% protein quality for flax (both based on limiting value, Lysine).

Flax has a strong, dominating flavor. ANUTRA® has a neutral flavor and will take on the flavors of whatever it is mixed with.

Flax contains substances called cyanogens, which are converted in the body into another chemical called Thyocyanate (SCN). High blood concentrations of SCN for prolonged periods of time may have adverse effects in the thyroid function. ANUTRA® contains no harmful cyanogens. Flax also contains vitamin B interrupters that can cause malnutrition. The US government regulates flax consumption to no more than 12% of your total caloric intake. Vegans and others on diets low in protein or sulfur-containing amino acids (methionine and cystine) must be very careful consuming flax seed. Flax seed cyanogens convert to cyanide, a poison that can be life threatening!

FDA has approved ANUTRA® (*Salvia Hispanica L*) as regular food. Flax is not FDA approved as a regular food and is illegal or restricted in some countries. Due to ANUTRA's® antioxidant and vitamin content, oxidation is minimal or non-existent. ANUTRA® does not require refrigeration.

WHY IS ANUTRA® BETTER THAN FLAX?

ANUTRA's® overall nutritional profile is far superior to flax or any other whole food plant or animal. ANUTRA® has 25% more protein, twice as much calcium, and 25 times more lignans than flax, plus more antioxidants than flax or cultivated blueberries. It's also the highest and safest natural source of Omega-3's, antioxidants, fiber and lignans. ANUTRA® has a neutral taste and does not require refrigeration. Whole or ground ANUTRA® digests beautifully while flax must be ground. ANUTRA® also has a unique gelling quality that works well in recipes. The FDA has approved ANUTRA® (*Salvia Hispanica L.*) as regular food like rice, corn, oats, wheat, soy bean, etc. Flax is not FDA-approved as a regular food and is illegal or restricted in some countries. Low protein diets with little methionine and cystine and dangerous toxins present in whole flax, may cause serious vitamin B interruptions, malnutrition and thyroid interruptions. Thyroid interruptions may cause a general deterioration of overall health and metabolism problems. Even a slightly under-active thyroid during pregnancy might trigger premature birth and babies born with lower IQs. During pregnancy, having sufficient thyroid hormones is essential for fetal-brain development and avoiding miscarriage or premature births.

ANUTRA® absorbs more than 15 times its weight in water. Flax absorbs only 6 times its weight in water. ANUTRA's® unique soluble fiber forms a gel in the stomach that creates a physical barrier between carbohydrates and the digestive enzymes that break them down. This process slows down the conversion of carbohydrates into sugar. ANUTRA® gels better than flax.

ANUTRA's® neutral flavor and its hydrophilic structure lends itself to limitless recipe applications.

CLINICAL STUDIES

Many of the health benefits of ANUTRA's® nutrient dense properties were validated through extensive acute and long-term studies conducted at the University of Toronto. In an acute study, after-meal blood glucose and plasma insulin levels were reduced thereby improving insulin sensitivity. In a long-term trial, blood pressure was reduced. High blood pressure is a major cardiovascular risk factor in those with Type 2 Diabetes.

In the same study, ANUTRA's® nutrient dense properties proved to be effective in reducing risk factors of heart disease, body inflammation, and coagulation factors ("aspirin-like effects"). These clinical results indicate the great potential of ANUTRA® as a functional food useful in the prevention and non-drug treatment of heart disease. ANUTRA's® extremely high content of Omega-3 fatty acids, Lignans and nutrient rich composition creates exceptional possibilities for the improvement of health and nutrition. Studies continue to reveal more of the vast benefits of this powerful grain and more exciting results are expected. ANUTRA® can be considered a perfect functional food.

Starting in the 1970's, researchers began to explore the importance of Omega-3's in our daily diet. Since then, numerous clinical studies conducted worldwide prove that Omega-3's are vitally important to our optimum health and will positively affect many of the common disorders and diseases we face today.

THE IMPORTANCE OF OMEGA-3 FATTY ACIDS

Omega-3 fatty acids are a form of polyunsaturated fat, one of the 4 types of fat that we get from the foods we eat (saturated fat, monounsaturated fat and trans fat are the others). All poly- and mono-unsaturated fats, including Omega-3's, are essential to our overall good health.

Many of us already know that eating foods high in saturated fat and trans fat are associated with the development of many diseases such as heart disease and cancer. Polyunsaturated and monounsaturated fats are the "good fats". Omega-3's along with Omega-6's, another type of poly-unsaturated fat, are essential fatty acids (EFA's). Our bodies do not make these important fats. We can only obtain EFA's from eating foods that contain them thus making the outside sources of these fats "essential". Omega-9's (Oleic Acid) are necessary but are non-essential since the body manufactures modest amounts.

Many of the foods we eat daily contain more Omega-6's than Omega-3's. Omega-6's are found naturally in cereals and whole grain breads. Omega-3's are found in ANUTRA® and in flax; in cold-water fish such as salmon, herring, sardines, tuna, mackerel and halibut; in dark green leafy vegetables; and in certain vegetable oils. Health experts agree that consuming a good ratio of these two EFA's is a vital key to optimum health.

Cold-water fish are not the highest or safest source of Omega-3's. It is now highly recommended that our fish consumption be limited to no more than two servings per week because of the health risks associated with ingesting the high dioxin (one of the most toxic chemicals known) and high, dangerous mercury levels these fish may contain. ANUTRA® is the highest and safest natural source of Omega-3's and Lignans known. There is virtually no chance of ingesting dangerous toxins or chemicals with ANUTRA®.

For most of our existence, we have eaten foods containing equal amounts of Omega-3's and Omega-6's in a ratio of 1:1 or with more Omega-3's in a ratio of 2:1. However, over the last 50 years our eating habits have changed. We generally consume Omega-6's to Omega-3's in a ratio of 20:1 and, depending on your diet, your Omega-6 intake can be as high as 50:1 over Omega-3's. The diet changes that have negatively impacted the important ratio of Omega-3's to Omega-6's are the inclusion of huge amounts of highly refined oils we use in cooking or in prepared foods. Examples of these are corn oil, safflower oil, cottonseed oil, peanut oil, and soybean (all high in Omega-6's).

ANUTRA® contains a ratio of 3:1 (3 Omega-3's to 1 Omega-6's) and this ratio is considered to be the best ratio of Omega-3's and Omega-6's. ANUTRA's® Omega-3 is called Alpha-Linolenic acid(ALA). ALA is critical to our health and well-being for so many reasons. One important factor is if the body does not have sufficient Omega-3's, it will use saturated fat to construct cell membranes.

ANUTRA® VS. FLAX

Serving Size:15 g	ANUTRA®	FLAX
Protein	4 g	3 g
Carbohydrates	5 g	6 g
Dietary Fiber	5 g	3 g
Omega-3's	3,000 mg	3,000 mg
Lignans	1,275 mg	>50 mg
ORAC	75 per g	61 per g
Vitamin E	764 mcg	18 mcg
B Vitamins	2,146 mcg	784 mcg
Vitamin C	< 375 mcg	75 mcg
Vitamin A	< 3 IU	NONE
Calcium	78 mg	30 mg
Selenium	11 mcg	4 mcg
Manganese	342 mcg	30 mcg
Chromium	11 mcg	NONE
Iron	1,007 mcg	750 mcg
Copper	240 mcg	150 mcg
Vitamin B Interrupter	NO	YES
Thyroid Interrupter	NO	YES
FDA Reg Food Approved	YES	NO

Source for ANUTRA®: Microbac Labs / Source for Flax: Flax Institute of the US(USDA SR19)

There are also two "non-essential" Omega-3's fatty acids. They are DHA (docosahexaenoic acid) and EPA (eicosapentaenoic acid), which the body makes from ALA and which are present in some fish oil.

Fish oil companies and others would like you to believe that the body's conversion process of ALA into DHA and EPA is not adequate because the high consumption of Omega-6's in the average American diet may slow the conversion of ALA into DHA and EPA; however, the high levels of vitamin B-6, zinc and magnesium found in ANUTRA® counter this charge and allows for proper conversion factors.

GOOD NEWS FOR OMEGA-3'S...

The USDA's food pyramid is currently revising its dietary guidelines to state that Omega-3's are beneficial to good health and trans fats are detrimental to good health.

The American Heart Association also recently revised its dietary guidelines to recommend consuming foods high in Omega-3's.

ANUTRA® is an easy and enjoyable way to eat more Omega-3's!

MORE ON WHY ANUTRA® IS SO "ESSENTIAL"

There are only two essential fatty acids that we MUST get from our diet because our body does not make them. They are:1. Alpha-linolenic Acid (ALA or LNA), an Omega-3 which is abundant found is ANUTRA® and 2. Linoleic Acid (LA) which is an Omega-6 also found in ANUTRA®.

Remember, they are essential because the body requires them for our life and good health. Consuming too few Omega-3's results in degenerative symptoms but eating sufficient amounts of Omega-3's can help reverse degenerative symptoms and bring us back to good health.

ANTIOXIDANTS

Antioxidants are substances or nutrients in our foods which have been shown to prevent or slow the oxidative damage to the cells in our bodies. Although supplementation is recommended for some individuals, the best method of obtaining antioxidants is through the diet. Whole foods have special quantities unmatched by mankind.

Antioxidants are found abundant in beans, whole grains, fruits, and vegetables. The use of oxygen by our bodies produces free radical by-products which can damage any cell, such as those in the heart, lungs, kidneys, brain, liver, musculoskeleton, and gastrointestinal tract. Antioxidants act as free radical scavengers and help to prevent and repair cellular injury. Conditions such as heart disease, cancer, diabetes, neurological disorders, and autoimmune diseases may all be potentiated by free radicals.

Recent studies have shown that consuming 9 servings of fruits and vegetables as recommended by the USDA per day will help to keep our bodies strong and healthy. ORAC values (oxygen radical absorption capacity) are being established for foods as a new and evolving concept for enabling researchers and consumers to measure daily consumption of antioxidants. Currently, there is no established daily RDA for ORAC in the US, although an average serving of fruits and vegetables is 2200 ORAC's; therefore 2200 times 9 servings per day equals approximately 20,000 ORAC's per day to be considered a healthy daily amount. ANUTRA® provides 75 ORAC units per gram (1,125 per serving).

ANUTRA's® ORAC value is ranked in the top 10 best foods for antioxidants- higher than cultivated blueberries or flax.

THE IMPORTANCE OF LIGNANS

Lignans are a type of phytonutrient (natural healing compounds) found in the cell matrix of certain seeds and grains including ANU-TRA®. When we ingest Lignans, they are broken down in the digestive track into two main Lignans-enterodiol and enteolactone. These Lignans circulate through the liver and subsequently are excreted in the urine. They mimic the hormone estrogen thereby blocking the formation of hormone-based tumors and growths. They are considered to be "phytoestrogens."

Lignans have numerous biological properties that make them unique and very useful in promoting good health and combating various diseases. These amazing compounds have shown such extraordinary potential that the National Cancer Institute has studied Lignans for their cancer preventative properties (for breast, colon and prostate-cancer) as well as for their anti-viral, anti-bacteria and anti-fungal effects. It has been concluded that the release of Lignans into the body blocks the action of some cancer-causing substances. Lignans are also a powerful antioxidant and have been shown to enhance the immune system. There is mounting scientific evidence showing how important it is to consume a Lignan-rich diet.

ANUTRA® has 8.5 grams of Lignans per 100 grams (3 1/2oz.) compared with approximately 0.3 grams per 100 grams of flax seed. ANUTRA® is the richest grain source of Lignans known.

WORLDS' FIRST GRAIN PROVEN TO REDUCE INFLAMMATION

Recent groundbreaking evidence indicates that the presence of "inflammation" in the body is as dangerous a health concern as high cholesterol in the development of arterial disease, heart attack and strokes. This "inflammation" is easily measured with a simple test that examines the level of a chemical called C-reactive protein (CRP), which increases dramatically during inflammation. CRP the marker for inflammation, is a molecule produced by the liver in response to an inflammatory signal that can come from arteries clogged with excess fat deposits or plaque. This occurs more frequently in people who are over-weight and obese.

Previous studies have associated people with elevated CRP levels to have a higher risk of experiencing heart attacks, strokes and Type 2 Diabetes. Experts have determined that having CRP levels of 0.5mg/l or less rarely have heart attacks. Other recent finding strongly indicate a relationship between higher CRP levels and the potential risk of colon cancer.

In randomized clinical studies, ANUTRA's® extraordinary profile of antioxidant vitamins, calcium, magnesium, other important vitamins and minerals and its rich levels of Omega-3's fatty acids proved to be effective in reducing inflammation levels and corresponding CRP levels in individuals with Type 2 Diabetes by 21%.

HUGE CALORIE SAVINGS WITH ANUTRA® !

Only 3-1/2 oz (100g) of ANUTRA® Provides us with

OMEGA-3'S (20G)	=	2 LBS OF ATLANTIC SALMON
VEGETABLE PROTEIN (24G)	=	1-1/2 CUPS OF KIDNEY BEANS
CALCIUM (520MG)	=	1-3/4 CUPS OF WHOLE MILK
FIBER (32G)	=	1-1/2 CUP OF ALL-BRAN
POTASSIUM (552MG)	=	1-1/4 BANANA
MAGNESIUM (231MG)	=	2-1/4 LBS OF BROCCOLI
IRON (6.7MG)	=	2 LBS. OF RAW SPINACH
519 TOTAL CALORIES		MORE THAN 3,000 TOTAL CALORIES

HEART HEALTH

Omega-3's are clinically proven to lower cholesterol and triglyceride levels, stabilize heart arrhythmia, lower blood pressure (reduces hypertension), act as a natural blood thinner thereby reducing the "stickiness" of blood cells and increase HDL ("good") cholesterol. Approximately 60% of the fat found in ANUTRA® is from Omega-3's with ALA (Alpha-Linolenic Acid) making it a very rich, natural source of Omega-3's.

COLORECTAL CANCER

Studies conducted at Johns Hopkins prove those with high levels of C-Reactive Protein (CRP) are 2.5 times more likely to develop colon cancer. Clinical studies also prove ANUTRA's® extraordinary profile reduces C Reactive Protein levels that in turn may help reduce the risk of colorectal cancer.

BREAST CANCER

Preliminary research at the University of California, Los Angeles suggests that Omega-3's may help maintain healthy breast tissue and prevent breast cancer. ANUTRA® may also promote healthier skin and hair.

PROSTATE CANCER

There have been a number of studies proving that diets high in Omega-3's and fiber may help reduce the risk of prostate cancer. A Duke University Medical Center pilot study concluded that even short-term changes to a high-fiber/Omega 3 supplemented diet resulted in prostate cancer cells that did not divide as quickly as those in men not on the diet. ANUTRA®, with its high Omega-3 and fiber content, is an easy and simple way to include these necessary nutritional benefits into your daily diet.

OSTEOPOROSIS

Per weight, ANUTRA® contains 6 times more calcium than milk. We need calcium to prevent bone loss. ANUTRA® is a rich source of the minerals phosphorous, magnesium and iron all of which aid in the absorption and utilization of calcium by the body. The concentration of protein in milk and dairy products in general decreases calcium absorption.

One can attain only 35% calcium absorption when consuming milk, while ANUTRA® allows an astonishing 85% calcium absorption when taken.

PRE-NATAL HEALTH

The American Journal of Clinical Nutrition reported that Omega-3's are very important to nourish the developing brain of the fetus and to the mental health of the mother. If the mother's intake of Omega-3's is minimal, the fetus will use all that's available. Research also shows this may cause depression in the mother. ANUTRA® is a rich, natural source of Omega-3's. ANUTRA® also contains essential amino acids, phytonutrients, vitamins and minerals including folate (folic acid) all of which are extremely important in pregnancy and in fetal development.

DEPRESSION AND OTHER MENTAL HEALTH PROBLEMS

The International Journal of Clinical Practice tells us that much research (including research from Harvard) has linked low levels of Omega-3's in the body with mood disorders. Omega-3's are believed to keep the brain's pattern of thoughts, reactions, and reflexes running cohesively and efficiently. Clinical trials have concluded that Omega-3's may reduce the risk of various psychiatric disorders and Alzheimer's disease.

HEALTHY WEIGHT LOSS

ANUTRA® can be a valuable tool for weight control when added to your favorite recipes. ANUTRA® is so nutrient dense that you would have to eat two pounds of Atlantic Salmon to get what you would in Omega-3's from just 100 grams of ANUTRA®. Many calories can be saved when ANUTRA® is used in recipes. Use in drinks, smoothies, cereal, yogurt, breads, pizza dough, muffins, pancakes, waffles, omelets, dressings, sauces, jams, deserts, and much, much more! Also, instead of having to eat fish all the time for the Omega-3's, try putting ground ANUTRA® into your favorite barbeque or steak sauce making your favorite lean meat more Omega-3 rich than any fish! Let your imagination go to incorporate ANUTRA®. In addition, ANUTRA's® exceptionally high level of Tryptophan (an amino acid that suppresses appetite) may positively affect satiety.

MENOPAUSE

ANUTRA® with its high Omega-3 and Lignan content, may enhance and balance hormone replacement therapy (HRT). ANUTRA® may help reduce hot flashes and other symptoms of menopause and help maintain a positive mental outlook.

HIGH QUALITY PROTEIN

For those who are on high protein diets, ANUTRA® provides 74% of its calories from lipids and high quality plant protein with very few calories from carbohydrates. The carbohydrates portion of ANUTRA® is predominantly insoluble fiber. Insoluble fiber, which is very beneficial to digestion, is a "non-carbohydrate" carbohydrate in that it passes through the gastro-intestinal tract undigested resulting in a non-caloric effect to our body.

The proteins in ANUTRA® show an excellent distribution of amino acids including all essential amino acids. Calculation of the Protein Efficiency Ratio (PER), or biological value, indicates ANUTRA's® protein has a digestibility in the range of other proteins used in nutritional products of the highest standard. The PER, or biological value for ANUTRA®, is slightly lower than that of casein, a skim milk protein and a standard of comparison of protein quality. However, it is slightly higher than that of soy protein, a common and highly regarded source of quality protein. Protein quality is the estimated percentage of protein that is likely to be used by the body. Protein quality calculations yield relative protein quality for ANUTRA® of 91% and for flax of 60% (both based on limiting value, Lysine)

AMINO ACIDS, VITAMINS AND MINERALS

ANUTRA® is a rich source of all essential amino acids and of antioxidant vitamins and minerals. It is very rich in calcium and iron; contains Vitamins A and C, potassium, phosphorous and magnesium, and is a good source of B vitamins including folic acid (60 mcg per 3 1/2oz.), an important B-vitamin especially needed for pre-natal health. ANUTRA® has 3 to 10 times the oil concentration of most grains and 1 1/2 to 2 times the protein concentration of other grains. These oils are the essential oils your body needs to help absorb the fat soluble vitamins A, D, E, & K.

FIBER & GASTRO-INTESTINAL HEALTH

Due to its high concentration of dietary fiber, ANUTRA® may help maintain optimum intestinal health. Approximately 32% of ANU-TRA® is fiber and of this amount nearly 100% of it is insoluble fiber. This is considerably higher than wheat bran and flax. Whole or ground ANUTRA® digests beautifully while flax must be ground. ANUTRA's® high fiber improves laxation, prevents occasional constipation and aids in colon cleansing*. You will notice a positive change in your bowel movement and stool. ANUTRA's® fiber helps maintain healthy bloodglucose and cholesterol levels*. Simple carbohydrates are digested in approximately 20 minutes in the first 2-4 feet of our intestinal tract. Our bodies tell our brain that it needs more food because of the rapid insulin-spike and fall created by eating simple carbohydrates. ANUTRA® contains a very special complex carbohydrate generally taking 3-4 hours to digest and utilizes 18-20 feet of our intestinal tract. This slower digestion period keeps your body hydrated longer and lets you fully absorb all of ANUTRA's® valuable nutrients thus dramatically increasing your energy and endurance.

ANUTRA® is also a hydrophilic colloid (a watery, gelatinous substance which forms the underlying elements of all living cells). This important property aids in the digestion of food and supports a healthy digestive tract*.

RHEUMATOID ARTHRITIS AND OTHER AUTOIMMUNE DISEASES

Since studies prove that Omega-3" help the arteries and other parts of the body stay inflammation free, it is believed that diets high in

Omega-3's increase survival for those with autoimmune diseases. Increasing your intake of Omega-3's may reduce the use of non-steroidal anti-inflammatory drugs (NSAID's)

VASODILATOR

Vasodilation occurs when the arteries are enlarged which improves circulation and oxygen transport. Due to its nutrient dense properties, ANUTRA® likely has a vasodilatory effect by increasing the size of the arteries and thereby lowering blood pressure. This is the same effect achieved by "Viagra(tm)"- type medication and should work the same for women as it does for men.

ATHLETES

ANUTRA®, a cornucopia for the 21st century, is the new version of "the running food" used by the ancient Aztecs and the Indians of the southwest. It was said that the Indians would eat as little as a teaspoon when going on a 24-hours forced march. The soluble fiber in ANUTRA® forms a gel in the stomach that creates a physical barrier between carbohydrates and the digestive enzymes that break them down. This process slows the conversion of carbohydrates into sugar. This stabilization of blood sugar creates endurance. ANUTRA® also holds 15 times its weight in water; thereby offering prolonged hydration. ANUTRA® helps us retain moisture and absorb our nutrients more efficiently resulting in electrolyte balance. ANUTRA's® high protein efficiency ratio helps regenerate muscle tissue and its clinically proven reduction of inflammatory markers increases physical performance and accelerates sports recovery.

TYPE 2 DIABETES

ANUTRA's® nutrient dense qualities have been clinically proven to significantly improve metabolic control of diabetes. In an acute study, after-meal blood glucose and plasma insulin levels were reduced thereby improving insulin sensitivity. In a long-term trial, blood pressure was reduced. High blood pressure is the major cardiovascular risk factor in those with Type 2 diabetes.

LACTIC ACID BUILD-UP

With physical exertion, especially in sports-related activities, lactic acid build-up can occur in the muscle and possibly cause cramping or burning. Muscle recovery time after exercise is decreased with the breakdown of lactic acid build-up. Due to its extraordinary high Omega-3/Amino Acid profile, ANUTRA® may affect lactic acid build-up because of its ability to reduce body inflammation.

ANUTRA® AS A GREAT "POTENTIATOR"

All of us who care about our family's and personal health, develop foods and other ways such as taking vitamins and other supplements to fortify our health and personal well-being. If you are anything like me, and the average American, you are consuming some functional foods and supplements. Many of us take a therapeutic aspirin a day and certain other vitamins and minerals as well as herbs to fortify our health. And we all know too well, as we get older, the medications we sometimes have to take. ANUTRA® has so many special qualities that it makes what you are presently taking work so much better. The aspirin and other supplements, like vitamins, minerals and

herbs, can affect your stomach and digestive tract. ANUTRA's®
unique digestive qualities and many helpful synergistic nutritional
factors enables the maximum benefits to be derived from whatever
supplement, vitamin, mineral, herb or prescription drug that you use.

ANUTRA® BENEFIT WITH MEDS AND VITAMINS

Many of us who take certain medications and vitamin supplement
may suffer from an irritation to the lining of our stomach that in turn
causes abdominal pain and discomfort. Additionally, medications
and vitamins may sometimes "get stuck" in our esophagus. Some
medications which are widely known to cause stomach discomfort are
NSAIDS such as aspirin, Advil, Aleve, Motrin and other well-known
NSAIDS brands, steroids, cholesterol lowering meds, high blood
pressure meds, cancer meds and many others.

ANUTRA® the world's healthiest whole food is a great potentiator.
A potentiator is a safe catalyst enabling foods, vitamins, minerals and
medications to to work better because their nutritional environment
has been significantly enhanced.

By taking your meds and vitamins with 2 tablespoons of ground or
whole ANUTRA® mixed with water, milk or juice (which hydrates
the ANUTRA®), you will dramatically reduce the risk of irritating
your stomach lining and prevent the possibility of them getting stuck
in your esophagus. ANUTRA's® unique soluble fiber content combined with its hydrophilic colloidal properties makes a gel in the
stomach that creates a physical barrier thereby "lining" the stomach
to prevent irritation caused by certain meds and vitamins.

THE ANUTRA® EXPLOSION

With all of the known healthy benefits of ANUTRA's® nutrient dense profile, we believe there is a wealth of other ANUTRA® health benefits yet to be discovered. The structural richness of this super grain makes it destined to become one of the most important foods of our lifetime to help improve our longevity and maintain our optimum health and well-being*.

ANUTRA's® unique composition offers a more nutritious alternative to other grains and its wonderful texture in gel form makes it easy to use as a baking ingredient and in many other ways. ANUTRA® may also be used in conjunction with almost any diet your doctor advises for your condition. At ValuHealth, we believe ANUTRA® will be recognized as one of the best proteins and one of the best overall nutrition sources in the world.

ANUTRA® GEL RECIPE

Anutra® gel is perfect for baking breads, pizza dough, muffins, pancakes, salad dressings, mayonnaise, nut butters, jams, jellies, gravies, puddings, desserts and much more. Approximately 5 ounces of Anutra® gel equals one 15g serving of ANUTRA®.

Adding Anutra® gel to any recipe gives the product a smooth texture while leaving the flavor intact. You have also displaced calories and fat by using Anutra® gel, an ingredient that is 90% water. For baked foods, you can substitute the oil in your recipes with Anutra® gel. For best results, decrease the recommended oil amount by 20% and replace this amount with Anutra® gel.

To make Anutra® gel use 9 parts of purified water to one part ANU-TRA® (by weight). One pound of ANUTRA® will make 10 pounds of Anutra® gel. Slowly pour ANUTRA® into water while briskly mixing with wire whisk, wait a few minutes and whisk again. Let the gel stand 5-10 minutes. Whisk the mixture again before storing into refrigeration. Anutra® gel will last 3 days in refrigeration. When baking and in breading's use 3 parts flour and 1 part ANUTRA®. In recipes, replace 1 egg with 1/4 cup Anutra® gel.

THE ANUTRASIZING™ DIET
A NEW YOU IN 90 DAYS!

Did you know that every 90 days your body regenerates nearly all its cells (7 to 10 trillion)? When you regenerate healthier, stronger, smoother, more elastic cells, you slow the normal aging process. Be the best you can be.

The Anutrasizing™ diet and exercise program makes it quick and easy to jump-start your healthy weight loss program. It will greatly increase your energy, stamina and overall wellness. Here is all you need to do:

BREAKFAST & LUNCH

Make an Anutrasizer™ (275 calories). Combine 6 oz. of your favorite Anutra® milk or healthy alternative and 6 oz. of fruit juice; add 3 tbsp. of whole grain ANUTRA® or 3 3/4 tbsp of ground ANUTRA®; stir until smooth (or just use 12 oz. milk). With your Anutrasizer™, eat either a banana (80 calories) and apple (90 calories) or 1 cup of strawberries (45 calories) and 1/2 cup of blueberries (40 calories).

You can also put 12 oz of milk in a blender, mix the same amount of ANUTRA® and add either a banana, an apple with ground cinnamon, or the strawberries and blueberries; blend all the ingredients until smooth.

Take a high-quality multi-vitamin with your Anutrasizer™ breakfast. This is not a necessity, but it does add nutritional assurances. Total calories for breakfast & lunch: approximately 750 calories. Drink at least 8 full glasses of water per day and drink one of these glasses after each Anutrasizer™.

DINNER

For women under 250 lbs., you can consume 450-500 calories at dinner for a total of 1,200 daily calories. For men under 250 lbs., you can consume 700 calories at dinner for a total of 1,400 calories. If you weigh over 250 lbs., please follow this chart for daily calories intake:

WEIGHT	CALORIE GOAL	
LBS.	WOMEN	MEN
250 or less	1,200	1,400
251-300	1,400	1,600
301 or more	1,600	1,800

Be sure to include 5 to 8 ounces of lean protein each day.

IMPORTANT NOTE: PLEASE CONSULT YOUR PHYSICIAN BEFORE STARTING ANY WEIGHT-LOSS PROGRAM.

MORE ON ANUTRASIZING™

Exercise (brisk walk, run, bike ride or other aerobic activity) at least 30 or more minutes per day preferably after your evening meal. Dieting alone can help you lose weight, but adding 30 or more minutes of aerobic exercise at least 4 days a week can double your rate of weight loss. After about 20 minutes of aerobic exercise, the body needs to use its stored fat as fuel. Therefore, the longer you exercise aerobically, the more calories you will burn. Strength training exercises such as weight training are also very important since they help counteract muscle loss due to aging. And, since calories are burned in muscle, muscle mass is a key factor in helping maintain a healthy weight. The more lean muscle mass you can preserve, the bigger "engine" in which to burn calories.

WHAT IS YOUR DESIRABLE WEIGHT?

Body Mass Index (BMI) relates to your body weight and to health risks associated with being overweight. To figure out your BMI, do the following calculation:

1. Multiply your weight in pounds by 0.45

(example- 150 lbs X 0.45= 68)

2. Multiply your height in inches by 0.025

(5 ft 10 in= 70 in X 0.025= 1.75)

3. Square your answer from step 2

(1.75 X 1.75= 3.0)

4. Divide your answer from step1 by the answer from step3

(68/3.0=22.6)

Your estimated BMI is 22.6. Generally, a healthy BMI ranges from 19 to 25. If your BMI is more than 25, talk with your physician about a weight-control program.

Remember to stay positive and stay with the program. Even if you have setbacks, persevering will get you where you want to be!

DOCTORS TALK ABOUT ANUTRA®

Significant Medical Data from

Dr. William J. Robbins M.D.

M.D.,F.A.C.P., A.A.H.I.V.S.
Diplomate, American Board of Internal Medicine
Diplomate, American Board of Internal Medicine Infectious Disease
Specialist, American Academy of HIV Medicine

"As a physician, I treat a significant number of immunocompromised patients. Secondary to their underlying disease, family history, medications, and lifestyle, the majority of my patients have significantly elevated triglycerides, total cholesterol, and LDL cholesterol (bad).

In addition, their good cholesterol (HDL) is low. Secondary to drug interactions with many of the statin drugs(Lipitor, Crestor, and others) need to be used and monitored extremely carefully as they can become potentially more toxic in these individuals. Even with the use of fibrates and fish oil or flax, getting to normal levels is impossible in the majority of my patients. Two a half years ago, I started taking ANUTRA® myself. Not only did my cholesterol level go to normal, but my HDL cholesterol increased significantly, and my LDL cholesterol decreased to normal levels. I decided to run the study on 32 of my patients. These patients were on a statin or fibrate, along with 3 -- 6 g of fish oil or the flax equivalent. Starting on 15 g (twotablespoons) of ANUTRA®, along with a decrease in the dose of their statin, and with the discontinuation of fish oil or flax, the average decrease in triglycerides was 132, total cholesterol decreased by 47, and bad cholesterol decreased by 15. These are all statistically significant. Those patients who took 15 g of ANUTRA® twice a day(4 tablespoons total) were able to discontinue all of their lipid lowering medications, some of my diabetics were able to discontinue their oral medications, and achieved the National Cholesterol Education Program (NCEP) guidelines and exceeded these guidelines. In addition, at 15 g twice a day, they all had significant increases in their HDL(good) cholesterol levels of between 10 and 40 points. Seeing what has occurred in them, many of them have their whole family and friends on ANUTRA®. It has no taste, mixes with anything, and actually saved them money because they do not have to buy statins, fibrates, fish oil, flax, nor any other pharmaceutical agents that are all very expensive. I truly recommend this to anyone who wants to live a healthy lifestyle, whether or not they have any other disease. In addition, ANUTRA® contains a healthy amount of fiber which is good for children and adults alike. I am a firm believer in ANUTRA® and will take it for the rest of my life." Many testimonial available on health wonders of ANUTRA® at www.anutra.com

Deborah F. Harding, M D

President and Founder of MD ONE ON ONE
Board Certified Internal Medicine
Board Certified Sleep Disorder Medicine
Diplomate of American Academy of Anti-Aging Medicine
Cenegenics Certified Age-Management Medicine

Dear Angelo:

Look at all the degenerative diseases with which we have to contend today. If we can do more to prevent those diseases early in life, patients are less likely to suffer them as they grow older. They're going to live longer and live better and have the ability to do things later in life that they were accustomed to doing in their youth.

After practicing traditional medicine for twenty-five years, I decided to do something radically different and offer more concentrated attention to the individual. I have renamed my Orlando, FL, practice: "MD One on One."

As a result, the patient's personal health care experiences have dramatically improved. Since preventive care and anti-aging have become my prime specialty, your product is helping every step of the way.

Because of poor dietary choices, most patients are Omega-3 deficient. I have found ANUTRA® to be the safest and most effective delivery system available for Omega 3's and other vital nutrients. It has a perfect ratio of Omega-3's, 6's and 9's, which are essential for good health. Deficiencies in DHA and EPA have been linked to serious health conditions, and adding ANUTRA® to your daily food intake should be a requirement in preventive medicine because the seven-to-ten trillion cells in your body are being regenerated every ninety days.

Quality of life and longevity are greatly enhanced through the maintenance of healthier, stronger, smoother, more elastic cells. The massive number of vital nutrients in ANUTRA® make it the singular most efficient method of delivery and I enthusiastically endorse your branding strategy: "nature's most perfect food." Having the major Omega-3 food source with a recommended daily allowance (RDA) from the Food and Drug Administration (FDA) is remarkable. The positive results in my patients have been astonishing.

They are sleeping better and awakening with more energy. They've never been more regular; constipation, diarrhea, bloating, gas and cramps disappear. Weight control becomes more manageable as hunger pangs and cravings vanish with a feeling of fullness. Their heart, arteries, blood pressure and cholesterol are behaving beautifully. Their joints feel more youthful with reduced stiffness. Their hair, skin and nails regain youthful luster. The evidence is overwhelming.

Rest assured that I take ANUTRA® and faithfully incorporate it into my family's daily nutrition as well.

Thank you, Angelo, for rediscovering this very important food source. Your perfect food product is fast becoming an absolute fountain of youth to aid my patients in fighting their aging battles.

Douglas A. Walsh, O.D.
Sports and Celebrity Physician Specialist

Hello, my name is Douglas A. Walsh, D.O. I am a family practice physician also specializing in sports medicine in Bradenton, FL, and surrounding areas. For over 38 years, I have been working with athletes on all levels of competition and in all sports. Most notably, I have worked for many years with professional baseball players who come to Florida for annual spring training.

I have recently found ANUTRA® to be a wonderful addition to an athlete's diet to help them achieve a higher level of performance in a number of ways. As we all know, maintaining hydration during workouts and sports activity is crucial. Because of ANUTRA's® soluble fiber and genetic make up, it swells to 15 times its weight in water and forms a gel in the stomach creating a physical barrier between the carbohydrates in the stomach and the digestive enzymes that break them down. This process slows the conversion of carbohydrate's into sugar.

Balancing carbohydrate absorption and stabilization of blood sugar allows your cells to get a slower, smoother supply of fuel providing sustained energy, electrolyte stability, endurance, and steady hydration.

I have also found that because of ANUTRA's® high protein efficiency ratio, antioxidants, and other vital nutrients, it is helping substantially in the recovery time for athletes from the standpoint of muscle soreness and reduced joint inflammation.

Understanding the importance of adding Omega 3's to the modern-day athlete's diet is essential. In today's sports, where split second decisions are the difference between winning and loosing, Omega 3's and their effect on an athlete's mental sharpness and cognitive abilities cannot be over stated.

Being mentally sharp and alert is what separates one physically gifted athlete from another; the difference between being good and great begins with the mind!

Medical science has learned that the greatest benefit of Omega 3's is that it replenishes and builds stronger, healthier cells, including muscle cells. Other than ANUTRA®, I know of no other major delivery source of omega 3's with an FDA Recommended Daily Allowance and regular food status.

In conclusion, I would strongly recommend that any serious athlete wanting to obtain maximum performance levels include ANUTRA® into their daily diet.

Here's to victory!

Dr. Wayne Coates
President of Anutra® Farms

Over the years as head of Arid Land Studies at the University of Arizona, I became familiar with many amazing plants, but nothing compares to my rediscovery of *Salvia Hispanica L.* Over 15 years ago, along with my colleague Ing. Ricardo Ayerza, we went to the keepers of the seed in Mexico. We then took the seeds and planted crops in many countries throughout the world. Over these years, I have been studying and utilizing new found knowledge to improve the grain without utilizing any genetically modification (Non-GMO).

The overall nutritional profile of this grain, now called ANUTRA®, is far superior to any food plant or animal. The Omega-3's, Omega-6's, Omega-9's and a small amount of necessary saturated fats are all in perfect alignment for optimum health. The antioxidants are of the highest quantities and are even higher than those found in cultivated blueberries. Also, ANUTRA® is very stable due to the high content of these antioxidants and unlike many other grains, especially flax, which oxidizes very quickly. When comparing the fiber content of the grain to others, ANUTRA® is much higher and contains both soluble and insoluble fiber that digests in a very special and healthy way. The lignans are very exciting because of their overall potential and particularly in their ability to possibly help in our quest to mitigate cancers. The overall protein of ANUTRA® is the highest of all grains or any other plant source and is more protein dense than chicken, turkey, fish, beef, pork, veal, lamb and other animal food sources.

I am very excited to continue my research and general improvement of *Salvia Hispanica L.* (ANUTRA®) as President of Anutra® Farms. I've accepted this position to further improve upon our understanding of this amazing food and to ensure the efficacy of this grain as we bring it to the world.

Part I

THE SEVEN SIMPLE STEPS
TO ANUTRASIZING™

STEP #1
Reduce your meat consumption by 10%.

There are three major reasons why you should reduce your consumption of meat by at least 10%. They are (1) your health and nutrition, (2) the environment, and (3) the world economy. For the purpose of what a 10% reduction would mean to you, I will assume you are consuming meat of some kind in two of your three meals each day. This would total approximately 14 meals each week that include meat. This is generally the case for most Americans. If this is so, I recommend that you start by eliminating at least two of these meals each week and replacing them with foods from plant proteins. Here are some of the reasons why:

HEALTH & NUTRITION

In the 1960's, scientists began suspecting that a diet high in animal fat is related to the development of arteriosclerosis and heart disease. Since that time, studies have scientifically shown that the consumption of animal fat, because of its relation to numerous serious maladies, is the greatest single cause of mortality in all developed countries of the world.

The human body is unable to deal with excessive amounts of animal fat and cholesterol. When we eat more cholesterol than the body needs (as we usually do with a diet high in animal fat), the excess cholesterol accumulates on the inner walls of the arteries. This may eventually lead to high blood pressure, heart disease, stroke, cancer, diabetes, and other diseases. Research strongly supports a link between high protein animal fat diets and cancer of the colon, rectum, breast, and uterus. These types of cancer are rare among those whose diets come primarily from plant proteins, such as the Japanese, Indians, and Seventh-Day Adventists.

On the flip side, scientists have continually proven that *plant proteins* may act to keep cholesterol levels low and help *prevent* heart disease, strokes, and certain cancers. Health statistics tell us that people living in nations eating primarily animal fats have a high cancer rate and people living in nations eating little or no animal fats have a minimal cancer rate.

Adding to these health issues is the alarming rise of obesity among adults and children. The rise in childhood obesity in particular is quite disturbing. You need only to think of how our children are predominantly being fed high-fat foods at quick-serve restaurants and are sitting for hours at their computers to know why this is the case. Portion sizes are out of sight, with burgers and french fries, which are high in saturated fat, being the normal meal of the day. Going out to play ball or other physical games with friends is becoming a thing of the past. Computer games are "in" these days. Adults are also exercising less and less and becoming heavier. If these trends continue, we are heading for a continued rise in coronary heart disease, cancer, diabetes, and other serious illnesses as well as exorbitant healthcare costs.

As our weight is going up, so are the cases of Type II diabetes, especially among children. There are now approximately 17 million people in the U.S. with the disease. According to the Department of

Health and Human Services, diabetes has increased 49% from 1990 to 2000 and projections indicate a 165% increase by the year 2050. If you have diabetes, you are at a very high risk for heart attack and stroke.

There is also a potentially dangerous health problem with the chemicals that are added to meat. As soon as an animal is slaughtered, its flesh begins to putrefy and becomes discolored. Adding nitrites, nitrates, and other harmful preservatives masks this discoloration. The meat then turns a bright red color. What most of us are not aware of is that many of these harmful preservatives are carcinogenic. And, as if the nitrites and nitrates aren't enough, the livestock are also given massive amounts of tranquilizers, hormones, antibiotics, and 2,700 other different drugs to keep them alive and fattened. These drugs are in the meat when you eat it, but the law does not require that they be listed on the packaging.

Another powerful reason why eating less meat will positively affect our health and nutrition is the recent EPA report on the significant amounts of cancer-causing dioxin found in meat. Dioxin concentrates in animal fat. The EPA tells us that Americans are getting 22 times the maximum dioxin exposure through their food and warns us to cut back on our consumption of meat and dairy products in which dioxin levels are highest. Dioxin is one of the most toxic organic chemicals known. It is defined as a family of 219 toxic chemicals found in the environment mostly as a by-product of ash from incinerators that have settled on crops eaten by livestock. In order to alleviate the problem, we have to tighten environmental controls and clean up the environment to reduce these highly toxic and persistent chemicals. This leads me to the next major reason why we should reduce our meat consumption.

THE ENVIRONMENT

The deterioration of the environment is another serious consequence of eating animal fat. The production of livestock creates ten times more pollution than residential areas and three times more than industry. The heavily contaminated runoff and sewage from slaughterhouses and feedlots are major sources of pollution in our rivers and streams. The fresh water resources of this planet are not only becoming contaminated but also diminished.

Water Scarcity and Pollution

I am sure you are aware of constant reports about our dangerously low water levels. I'll bet you didn't know that reducing your meat consumption would positively impact this serious threat.

Nearly half of the total amount of water used annually in the U.S. is used to grow feed and provide drinking water for livestock. U.S. fresh water reserves have significantly declined because of this, and water shortages, especially in the West, are at critical levels. In California, where 42% of irrigation is used for livestock feed or production, water tables have declined so low that in some areas the earth is sinking.

Consider the following fact: to grow one pound of wheat requires only 60 gallons of water, whereas production of one pound of meat requires anywhere from 2,500 to 6,000 gallons of water! As far back as 1973, the *New York Post* uncovered a shocking misuse of this most valuable resource - one large chicken slaughtering plant was using one hundred million gallons of water daily, an amount that could supply a city of twenty-five thousand people.

According to the Environmental Protection Agency (EPA), livestock waste has polluted 35,000 miles of rivers in 22 states and contaminated groundwater in 17 states, and 218 million people in the U. S. live within 10 miles of a polluted river, lake, stream, or coastal area. The EPA estimates that at least a half-million cases of illness annually can be attributed to contaminated drinking water. Uses of lagoons and a system called sprayfield, are the most common methods used by farmers to dispose of animal waste. Lagoons at many farms break, fail, or overflow spilling many thousands of gallons of waste into rivers, lakes, and streams. Farm operators using the sprayfield method spray waste into windy and rainy weather, on frozen ground, or on land already saturated with manure. The environmental impact from run-offs can be severe since manure is often over-applied or misapplied to cropland and pastures. The EPA's proposed technology rules relating to polluted lagoons do very little, if anything, to alleviate or solve this serious problem.

Global Warming - CO_2 Emissions

Beef production is also a significant factor in the emissions of three of the four global warming gases - carbon dioxide, nitrous oxide, and methane. Carbon dioxide is released into the atmosphere when forests are burned to make additional grazing land. It is also generated by fuel used in the highly mechanized agricultural production of feed crops for livestock. Fertilizers used to produce feed crops for grain-fed cattle release nitrous oxide, another greenhouse gas.

Nitrous oxide now accounts for 6% of the global warming effect. Cattle emit methane through belching and flatulation. Scientists estimate that more than 500 million tons of methane are released each year and that the world's more than one billion cattle and other livestock emit approximately 60 million tons, or 12% of the total from all sources. Methane is a serious problem because one molecule traps twenty-five times more solar heat than a molecule of CO_2.

Soil Erosion and Desertification

Livestock overgrazing and the burden that the grain used to feed the livestock puts on the land cause soil erosion and desertification. Over-cultivation and improper irrigation techniques are also principal causes. In the American West and in other parts of the world, what was productive land is turning into barren desert due to cattle grazing. Cattle farmers also degrade the land by stripping vegetation and compressing the earth.

A 1991 United Nations report stated that as much as 85% of U.S. rangeland (nearly 685 million acres) is being degraded by overgrazing and other problems. The study estimates that 430 million acres in the American West are suffering a 35% to 50% yield reduction largely because of overgrazing. That report was released more than ten years ago, so imagine what these figures are now.

Deforestation

Beef consumption is a significant cause of the destruction of the world's rainforests. Because it is such a lucrative business, ranchers burn rainforests to create new rangelands. In about a year or two, grazing quickly destroys rainforest soil and the ranchers move on to burn another rainforest area. It is a never-ending cycle of destruction. Many of us are not aware of why rainforests are so important to our very existence. Here are some important reasons why they are:

- 50% of the earth's oxygen is generated by rainforests;

- 50% - 90% of all life forms exist in the rainforest;

- Only 6% of the earth's land area is rainforest, yet 80% of all surface vegetation is in the rainforest;

- Rainforests are disappearing at an average rate of 100,000 acres a day; at that rate they will be totally destroyed in 30 - 50 years;

- 17% - 20% of the carbon dioxide introduced into the earth's atmosphere comes directly from the burning of rainforest;

- The "slash and burn" method of farming eventually eliminates the possibility of regeneration of vegetation by destroying seeds;

- 50% of ALL pharmaceuticals originated as plants with 25% of medicines still using plant extracts, yet less than 1% of rainforest plants have been screened for medical use;

- 70% of current medicines believed to have cancer-fighting properties are from the rainforest;

- We are losing an estimated 270 species a day to extinction - the fastest rate since the ice age.

Beef typically used by fast food hamburger chains or in processed beef products come from the rainforest. The U.S. imports over 200 million pounds of fresh and frozen inexpensive beef from Central American countries, where ranchers have already cleared two-thirds of their rainforests for cattle grazing. The FDA does not require that the beef be labeled with its country of origin. Because of that, a consumer does not know where it comes from. Reducing your consumption of beef, even by just 10%, will reduce demand for it, and cut back on pressure to clear more forests for cattle. Now, let's learn how cutting back on your meat consumption can help the world economy.

WORLD ECONOMY

There are many in the world who go hungry just so that meat demand can be met. To supply beef to the U.S., Europe, and Japan, beef cattle and their grazing land takes up nearly a quarter of the land mass. For the sake of producing meat, grain that could feed people is used to feed livestock instead. According to information compiled by the U.S. Department of Agriculture (USDA), over 90% of all the grain produced in America goes to feed livestock that ends up on dinner tables. We also use high protein grain from third world countries to feed our livestock; yet the process of using grain to produce meat is incredibly wasteful. For every 17 pounds of grain fed to cattle, we get back only one pound of meat.

In underdeveloped countries, a person consumes an average of four hundred pounds of grain a year, most of it by eating it directly. In contrast, the average American and European goes through two thousand pounds per year by first feeding almost 90% of it to animals. When there are more than a billion people in the world who lack food, I believe this is a grave social injustice. The beef industry will argue that this is feed grain, not food grain; however, the resources used to grow feed grain can very easily be used to grow food grains.

It is reprehensible that millions of people in third world countries are going hungry while their land, labor, resources, and plant-enriched proteins are being used to supply meat to the wealthy all over the world. Humankind can achieve many great things, but our ignorance of these facts and our greed do not allow us to see the truth. If Americans would reduce meat consumption by just 10%, enough grain would be saved to feed the 60 million people who die from hunger each year. Please think about this. If more people in the world were not hungry, they would be happier and more productive. Economically, the world would become more stable.

CONCLUSION

What we must understand is the solution to better health and nutrition, a cleaner and safer environment, and a more stable world is very simple - eat more plant proteins!

You can well imagine that just by following step one of ANUTRA-SIZE™ (reducing your meat consumption by 10%) you will be significantly impacting your physical well-being, while doing your part to ease the serious environmental and economic world problems we face.

As I said at the beginning of this chapter, I am recommending that you start with a mere reduction of 10% of your meat intake, perhaps only two of your meat meals each week. These meals should be replaced with foods from plant-proteins. I am hopeful that after reading these major life reasons to reduce meat consumption, you will decide to reduce your meat intake even more.

STEP #2
ANUTRA® MILK

Nature's Healthiest and Best Tasting!
(Plant or Animal)

"There is no reason to drink cow's milk at any time in your life. It was designed for calves, not humans, and we should stop drinking it today."

Dr. Frank A. Oski
Former Director of Pediatrics,
Johns Hopkins University

In the Bible, Exodus 3:8 tell us that the Israelites will be brought to a good and spacious land, a land flowing in milk and honey. Does this mean that we should drink cow's milk? I don't think so. My interpretation would be that the land the Israelites would be brought to would be a prosperous land, rich in resources, and where living beings were healthy and thriving. But, what if we were to take the "land of milk and honey" literally?

The honey from the bee is unadulterated and totally safe for our direct consumption, but today cow's milk is very adulterated. Even before it became so adulterated, I do not believe it was meant for human consumption. I concur with Dr. Oski, that cow's milk was intended for calves, not humans. Then why do humans drink the milk of another mammal? Do you think nature intended for us to do that? Why would it when human mothers are given their own milk producing means to nourish their young? Would we give a human mother's milk to an animal? Do different animals drink one another's milk? No, they do not. Cows produce milk to feed *their* young as do other mammals; therefore, injecting them with antibiotics, growth hormones, and other harmful chemicals places not only their young at risk, but also humans who consume it. Would you feed milk like that to your baby? Of course you wouldn't. But that is exactly what you are drinking if you drink cow's milk.

We already know that cow's milk is high in saturated fat and cholesterol. It also contains no fiber and no complex carbohydrates. Cow's milk has naturally occurring lactose, a milk sugar that is indigestible by more than 70% of the world's population. The prevalence of lactose intolerance varies by race and ethnicity with African Americans, Hispanics, and Asians the most effected. Allergic symptoms include abdominal bloating, gaseousness, flatulence, cramping, and diarrhea. Growth hormones and the numerous antibiotics given to cows can cause additional health problems. Even the great pediatrician, Dr. Benjamin Spock, once America's leading authority on child-care, spoke out against giving infants and children cow's milk, saying it causes anemia, allergies, insulin-dependent diabetes, and will eventually lead to obesity and heart disease.

About a decade ago, the FDA approved the use of a genetically engineered hormone called recombinant bovine growth hormone (rBGH). The purpose of injecting cows with this hormone is to increase the cows milk output. With our already enormous consumption of milk, economic justification for using the growth hormone is perplexing. The use of rBGH causes cows udders to become so painful and heavy (a condition called mastitis), their udders can literally drag on the ground. You will be more shocked to learn that laboratory studies have proven that animals treated with rBGH-developed cancer, yet the FDA will not reconsider their approval of the hormone.

There is another potentially dangerous hormone found in cow's milk called insulin-like growth factor-1 (IGF-1). Levels of this powerful hormone increase in the human body after milk consumption. In the past few years, IGF-1 has been named as a key factor in the angiogenesis and rapid metastasizing of various cancers including prostate, lung, and breast cancer. It is scientifically proven that this hormone survives digestion and encourages cells to grow - good ones and bad ones! In other words, it can find an existing cancer and signal it to grow. The IGF-1 hormone is an identical match between human and cow. Drink cow's milk or eat its cheese and you will ingest the dangerous IGF-1 hormone into your body.

Now, let's talk about calcium and cow's milk and the misleading information that it helps to prevent osteoporosis. Calcium intake is very important for our health; however, we do not have to drink gallons of cow's milk and consume loads of other dairy products to achieve proper calcium intake. Every cell in the body needs calcium to function properly. The heart, nervous system, and muscles all need calcium for their activity. Bones need calcium to maintain strength. Ninety-nine percent of body calcium is in the bones. You will be surprised to learn that important studies have shown that the more animal fat we eat, the more calcium we in fact *lose* and the more plant protein we eat, the *stronger* our bones become.

You may or may not be aware that many Asian countries, such as China and Japan, where dairy products are minimally consumed, have far less occurrences of osteoporosis than the U.S., where the average American consumes 40% of their annual bulk food from dairy products. The reasons their bones are stronger than Americans are simple. They eat far less animal fat, eat more vegetables, and they get more physical exercise. You can get enough calcium from eating certain vegetables and nuts without getting all of the harmful components of cow's milk in your system.

Several important studies have proven exactly the opposite of what the dairy industry wants us to believe. The higher your calcium intake from dairy products, the much greater your risk is for bone fractures. Again, this is because animal fat *causes* calcium depletion. Think about this telling fact. The countries that consume the most dairy products are Finland, Sweden, the United States, and England. The countries that have the highest rates of osteoporosis are Finland, Sweden, the United States, and England.

ANUTRA® MILK, nature's alternative milk from the plant kingdom, is a great tasting and highly nutritious milk made from ANUTRA®.

Serving for serving, ANUTRA® is more nutritious than cow's milk providing healthier protein, more calcium that will be properly absorbed by the bones, iron, and vitamins A, B, C, D, and E (antioxidants). It also contains just the right amount of monounsaturated and polyunsaturated fats, folic acid, and unlike cow's milk, which contains no fiber, Anutra® Milk contains valuable soluble and insoluble dietary fiber. It has no saturated fat, no trans-fatty acids, and is lactose free. ANUTRA® MILK taste and texture makes it perfect to use the same way you would use cow's milk; that is, for drinking or in recipes, and it's much better for you.

ANUTRA® MILK provide us with powerful phytonutrients, the beneficial chemical compounds naturally found in plant foods. These compounds have shown ANUTRA® provides us with powerful phytonutrients, the beneficial chemical compounds naturally found in plant foods. These compounds have been shown to be helpful in preventing a variety of diseases including many forms of cancer. It seems that phytonutrients promote the function of bodily enzymes that detoxify and suppress carcinogens and act as a protective measure against cell damage by optimizing our own natural defenses. There is no doubt that with the pesticides in our food, our air and water pollution, and the numerous other toxins we are exposed to each day, we need as much protection as we can get. By using the benefits of the phytonutrients found in plants, we can optimize our health and boost our preventative powers.

So, Anutra® Milk, with important phytonutrients and fiber, no saturated fat, no trans-fatty acids, no lactose, more absorbable calcium, essential vitamins, and other important minerals, is *much* better for us than cow's milk. Unlike cow's milk, toxin-free Anutra® Milk does not contain any dangerous growth hormones or antibiotics. At ValuHealth, we blend Anutra® Milk the same way we blend all of our products using a proprietary "hot process" which is guaranteed to eliminate the risk of dangerous pathogens such as E.coli, salmonella, and listeria. After learning all of this, which would you rather drink - Anutra® Milk or cow's milk?

Anutra® Milk vs. Cow's Milk

Nutrient	Anutra®	%DV/ %RDA	Whole Milk*	%DV/ %RDA
Calories	110		150	
Fat Calories	20		72	
Total Fat	2.5 g	4 %	8 g	12.5 %
Saturated Fat	0 g	0 %	5 g	25 %
Monounsaturated Fat	0.5 g		2.5 g	
Polyunsaturated Fat	1 g		0.5 g	
Cholesterol	0 mg	0 %	33 mg	11 %
Sodium	130 mg	5 %	120 mg	5 %
Total Carb	13 g	4 %	8 g	3 %
Fiber	2 g	10 %	0 g	0 %
Sugar	8 g		12 g	
Protein	9 g		8 g	
Vitamin A	1000 IU	25 %	307 IU	6 %
Vitamin C	15 mg	25 %	0 mg	0 %
Calcium	400 mg	40 %	291 mg	30 %
Vitamin D	120 IU	30 %	100 IU	25 %
Vitamin E	7.5 IU	25 %	0 IU	0 %
Iron	1.08 mg	6 %	0.12 mg	0 %
Phosphorus	230 mg	22 %	228 mg	22 %
Potassium	430 mg	12 %	370 mg	10 %
Riboflavin (B_2)	0.4 mg	23 %	0.395 mg	23 %
Vitamin B_6	0.5 mg	25 %	0.102 mg	5 %
Vitamin B_{12}	1.5 µg	25 %	0.871 µg	14 %
Folic Acid	100 µg	25 %	12 µg	8 %

Anutra® Milk Has:

Less Calories   More Vitamins A, C, D, E, B_6, B_{12}
No Saturated Fat More Calcium & Iron
No Cholesterol   More Folic Acid
More Protein   More Antioxidants
More Fiber   More Omega-3's and Lignans

SPECIAL NOTE:

LOOK FOR
ANUTRA®
DAIRY ALTERNATIVES

THE WORLD'S
HEALTHIEST
AND
BEST TASTING COMPLETE
LINE OF
DAIRY ALTERNATIVES

AVAILABLE LATER PART OF
2009.

**MEANTIME USE HEALTHY LOW-FAT DAIRY
AND DAIRY ALTERNATIVES**

STEP #3
Replace regular dairy products with
ANUTRA® BRAND DAIRY ALTERNATIVES
or other healthy alternatives

"Let your food be your first medicine."

Hippocrates, 337 BC

It is believed that cheese was first developed during prehistoric times more than five thousand years ago. Many food historians credit its discovery to an Arab nomad journeying across the desert. For his journey, the nomad carried milk in a leather pouch made from a sheep's stomach. When he stopped to drink the milk, he found that it had been turned into curds and whey by the combination of the hot sun and the rennet in the sheep's stomach. The first *record* of cheese dates back to around 3500 BC when the Sumerians are known to have made cheese. The Greek poet Homer also mentions cheese in the 9th century BC epic, the *Odyssey*. By the time of the Romans, cheese making became an art and this art has remained the same for most of history. The problem is that this "art" is not without its health risks.

Today, most cheese producers use stainless steel vats and pasteurize the milk before processing it into cheese. The milk is cooled to 85° at which point varied strains of bacteria and enzymes are added to separate the curds from the whey. Once this occurs, and depending on which type cheese is being made, the curd is pressed and aged for several days or months before the product is ready for consumption. This is a very expensive and time-consuming cold process in which there are many potential problems. At 85°, the milk is a rich blend of protein, fats, sugars, vitamins, and minerals. Dangerous pathogens such as E.coli, salmonella, listeria, streptococci, and many others, generally thrive in this type of environment and the presence of these pathogens in any food can cause many serious health problems. Additionally, the disposal of the separated whey, which is an abundant by-product of the cold cheese making process, is an environmental hazard which causes pollution.

Considering that 70% of our meals contain some form of dairy product, it is therefore very important we switch these dairy products with more nutritious **ANUTRA® BRAND DAIRY ALTERNATIVES**. The process we use to make **ANUTRA® BRAND DAIRY ALTERNATIVES** is a much safer process than the one I just described to you. We use a "hot" process that eliminates virtually any chance of dangerous pathogens. It is a process in which there is no expensive aging method and no pollution threat since we have no whey by-products. **ANUTRA® BRAND DAIRY ALTERNATIVES** have no saturated fat, cholesterol, or lactose so switching from conventional dairy products to ANUTRA® products can help eliminate the health risks and health costs associated with eating dairy products high in saturated fat and cholesterol.

Saturated fats are the very unhealthy fats. They make the body produce more cholesterol that may raise blood cholesterol levels. Excess saturated fat is linked to an increased risk of cardiovascular disease.

Of all the fats, saturated fat is the most powerful contributing factor of blood cholesterol levels. Saturated fats stimulate the production of LDL ("bad") cholesterol and therefore increase blood cholesterol levels and the risk of heart disease. In a 6 ounce chunk of full-fat cheddar cheese, there are 54 grams of saturated fat and 180 milligrams of cholesterol! **ANUTRA® BRAND DAIRY ALTERNATIVES contain *no* saturated fat, *no* trans-fatty acids, and *no* cholesterol.**

Healthy Omega-3's, antioxidants, fiber and lignans in ANUTRA® produces the world's healthiest milk.Monounsaturated and polyunsaturated fats are healthy fats since they do not promote the production of LDL ("bad") cholesterol but instead stimulate HDL ("good") cholesterol. They help *reduce* your risk of high cholesterol and coronary heart disease. Full-fat dairy products contain very little, if any, of these healthy fats. On the contrary, **ANUTRA® BRAND DAIRY ALTERNATIVES contain 3 grams of health-promoting mono- and polyunsaturated fats that help lower cholesterol.** In fact, if you put a Anutra® Slice on your hamburger, or Anutra® Shreds on your beef or chicken tacos, or pepperoni pizza, you can neutralize the effect of the LDL ("bad") cholesterol you are getting from the saturated animal fat with the HDL ("good") cholesterol-lowering mono- and polyunsaturated fats found in **ANUTRA® BRAND DAIRY ALTERNATIVES.** I call this "ANUTRA® Mathematics"; meaning any combination of an animal protein product with a **ANUTRA® BRAND DAIRY ALTERNATIVE** product equals a better formula for a healthier lifestyle.

Remember in the last chapter I told you about the numerous growth hormones and antibiotics that are given to cows and the health risks associated with these injections? I also told you about the dangerous hormone called insulin-like growth factor-1 (IGF-1) that is found in cow's milk. Well now we should think beyond the milk with regard to growth hormones, antibiotics, and IGF-1. These harmful hormones and antibiotics are in the cow's milk that is used to produce the cheese. Therefore, you can ingest these potentially cancer causing stimulants not only by drinking cow's milk, but also by eating dairy products made from cow's milk. **ANUTRA® BRAND DAIRY ALTER-NATIVES are made with wholesome ingredients and contain no growth hormones or antibiotics. They are toxin-free.**

In chapter one on reducing our meat consumption, I talked about how we must clean up the environment to reduce the highly toxic chemicals caused by certain industrial processes such as the manufacturing of some pesticides, smelting, and bleaching paper pulp. Dioxins are a by-product of some of these processes. They are among the most toxic substances on earth. Dioxins concentrate in animal fat and so meat and dairy products are considered the biggest dioxin sources. **ANUTRA® BRAND DAIRY ALTERNATIVES naturally have no dangerous dioxins.**

Dairy products from cow's milk also contain lactose. When you are lactose intolerant, you do not produce enough of the enzyme lactase that breaks down lactose in the small intestine. Lactose, or milk sugar, is a disaccharide composed of glucose and galactose. As I mentioned in chapter two, it is widely agreed that around 70% of the world's population is lactose intolerant. Symptoms include bloating, stomach pains, diarrhea, and flatulence. The incidence of lactose intolerance is especially rising in the aging population. As we get to be around fifty years of age, our ability to digest lactose sharply decreases. **ANUTRA® BRAND DAIRY ALTERNATIVES contain no lactose.**

When cows graze naturally from organic farmland where no pesticides are used, when they are treated humanely, and when they are not injected with harmful growth hormones or antibiotics, their milk is safe for their young. Cow's milk produced under these natural grazing conditions gives us a terrific by-product called casein. Unfortunately, organic and free-range farming is not practiced enough in the United States. It is much more widely practiced in Europe.

Casein, a highly nutritious skim milk protein with naturally occurring minerals, is extracted from skim milk in its pure form. It is widely used today as a nutritional and functional ingredient in dairy products. Casein contains 21 amino acids and has no saturated fat, cholesterol, or lactose. At ValuHealth, some of our ANUTRA® BRAND DAIRY ALTERNATIVES contain casein for its health benefits and its emulsifying function. The casein comes *only* from free-range cows that graze naturally. They are not given any harmful growth hormones or antibiotics and are therefore toxin free. You are getting pure casein in some ANUTRA® BRAND DAIRY ALTERNATIVES, which is beneficial to your health. It is the only dairy component found in some of our ANUTRA® BRAND DAIRY ALTERNATIVES and it is one we highly endorse. It is important to make you aware of this because there are some (very few) people who have milk allergies who may be allergic to casein. Certain milk allergies can be different than lactose intolerance. There are some types of casein, such as technical acid, hydrolyzed, lactic, and rennet that are used as commercial bonding agents. Please do not confuse these with the nutritious edible casein that is used in ANUTRA® BRAND DAIRY ALTERNATIVES.

For many of the same important reasons you would want to drink Anutra® Milk instead of cow's milk, you will want to eat ANUTRA® BRAND DAIRY ALTERNATIVES instead of full-fat dairy products. ALL ANUTRA® BRAND DAIRY ALTERNATIVE CONTAIN POWERFUL PHYTONUTRIENTS.

In summation, the important reasons to switch from conventional dairy products to ANUTRA® BRAND DAIRY ALTERNATIVES are the following:

More nutritious than conventional dairy products

Low fat - No saturated fat

Less Calories

Cholesterol and Lactose free

Trans-fatty Acid free

Reduce the risk of coronary heart disease, cancer, diabetes & other serious maladies

No harmful growth hormones or antibiotics

No harmful Dioxins

No dangerous IGF-1 hormone

Virtually no chance of E.coli, salmonella, listeria or other dangerous pathogens

Contains powerful healing and preventative phytonutrients like Omega-3's, antioxidants, fiber and lignans

Functionally equivalent in recipes to conventional dairy products

Sociologically the better choice

STEP #4
Eat a low-fat diet with no more than 25% of your total daily caloric intake derived from fats. Avoid saturated fat and trans-fatty acids (hydrogenated oils).

> Fat is "animal tissue consisting chiefly of cells distended with greasy or oily matter."
>
> Webster's Dictionary

How about that definition of fat! It sounds very much like something we want to avoid. Without hesitation, health experts agree that there is **too much fat** in the typical American diet. Scientific research strongly supports that this harmful excess fat is increasing our risk of heart disease, diabetes, and cancer of the prostate, colon, and breast. Numerous health and governmental authorities including the U.S. Surgeon General, the National Academy of Sciences, the American Heart Association, and the American Dietetic Association, advocate reducing dietary fat calories to 30% **or less** of total calories.

On average, Americans are consuming approximately 40% of their total calories from fat. Health professionals will tell you they would be thrilled if we would simply reduce the fat in our diets to around 30% of our total calories. They will also tell you that it is **far better** to have a diet in which **25% or less** of our total calories are derived from fat. Ten percent or less of our daily calories from fat may come from saturated fat. Ideally, if a person requires 1600 calories per day to maintain their perfect weight, their total daily fat intake should be approximately 40 to 45 grams with no more than 4 to 4.5 grams of the these fat grams coming from saturated fats.

Eating is a source of pleasure for many of us and is an important part of our lives. The food we eat sustains us, gives us energy, makes us grow, and helps heal our bodies. Within the foods we eat, there are different types of nutrients. Nutrients are classified into five major food groups: proteins, carbohydrates, fats, vitamins, and minerals. It is the types and amounts of proteins, carbohydrates, and fats we eat that will determine our health as well as our body weight and mass.

Proteins are the building blocks used to repair and grow our bodies. From the previous chapters, we have already learned that animal protein is typically high in saturated fat. Saturated fat is the harmful fat of which too much of in our diet can lead to our being overweight or obese. Therefore, it is much better to get most of our protein from plant-based foods that contain the healthier mono- and polyunsaturated fats.

There are two types of carbohydrates: simple and complex. Carbohydrates provide us with the power needed to fuel our bodies. Simple carbohydrates are sweet to the taste while complex carbohydrates are pleasant tasting, but not sweet. The healthiest complex carbohydrates are high-fiber vegetables, such as lettuce and broccoli, and low-fiber complex carbohydrates such as bananas, tomatoes, squash, and all cereal and grains. After digesting either simple or complex carbohydrates, they appear in our circulatory system in the form of glucose, which our cells utilize as energy. The high-fiber complex carbohydrates should be consumed in proper proportion for maximum health benefits. They contain rich sources of vitamins and minerals as well as important enzymes when they are in their raw state. The problem with carbohydrates is that when we alter them through processes they are stripped of their nutritional value and become "empty" calories.

Protein and carbohydrates provide about 4 calories per gram. Fat contributes more than twice as much — approximately 9 calories per gram. Fats store the energy we derive from our foods. Although there are fewer types of fats than carbohydrates, fats produce more than twice as much energy as carbohydrates. Being a compact fuel, fat is efficiently stored in the body for later use when carbohydrates are in short supply. Fats are necessary, but only in small amounts. They are important for growth and repair, to safeguard our bones and internal organs, and to provide some insulation against the cold.

We also need fats to transport lipid-soluble vitamins into the body. Lipid-soluble vitamins include A, D, E, and K, and they are not water-soluble. Some other lipids also serve the function of helping blood clot and helping the transmission of nerve pulses throughout the body. Cholesterol makes our skin and hair smooth, preventing them from becoming dry, and helping in the formation of Vitamin D.

But, it's the types of fats we eat and the total we consume each day that will make us healthy or unhealthy. Remember, we need to take in very little saturated fat (less than 10% of our daily recommended fat intake of 25%) and should get most of our 25% daily calories from fat through monounsaturated and polyunsaturated fats.

As many of us already know, fats are divided into two categories: saturated fats and unsaturated fats. Saturated fats, as we have previously discussed, are the "bad" fats. We need them only in very minimal amounts. Too much saturated fat can raise blood cholesterol levels and increase the risk for heart disease and certain cancers. We ingest saturated fats primarily from animal sources such as meat, cheese, and milk.

The unsaturated or "good" fats are monounsaturated and polyunsaturated fats. Monounsaturated fats tend to lower our LDL ("bad") cholesterol, elevate our HDL ("good") cholesterol, and reduce our triglyceride levels. Polyunsaturated fats supply essential fatty acids that the body does not make but can only get from food. Essential fatty acids are needed for normal growth, healthy skin, and they are vital to the brain and the nervous system. They also produce a hormone-like substance that helps regulate blood pressure, blood clotting, and the immune system.

There is another type of fat that we must try to totally avoid. It is a man-made fat which forms when vegetable oils are hydrogenated. Hydrogenation is a process that makes a liquid fat become solid at room temperature. The fat is called trans-fatty acid and it is found in many foods including margarine and shortening, fried foods such as french fries, and in cookies, donuts, crackers, and many other common processed foods. Trans-fatty acids raise LDL ("bad") cholesterol levels and may also lower HDL ("good") cholesterol in the blood. We need to minimize our intake of trans-fatty acids as well as saturated fats. **ANUTRA® BRAND DAIRY ALTERNATIVES have no trans-fatty acids.**

Here are some sources of good and harmful fats:

Good Fats	Harmful Fats
Monounsaturated Fats:	**Saturated Fats:**
Canola Oil	Dairy Products
Olive Oil	Beef, Chicken, Pork, Veal and all other meats
Peanut Oil	Coconut Oil
	Palm Kernel Oil
Polyunsaturated Fats:	Lard
ANUTRA® Oil	
Sesame Oil	**Hydrogenated Vegetable Oils:**
Safflower Oil	Man-made trans-fatty acids found in fried foods,
Corn Oil	cookies, crackers, doughnuts and more
Soybean Oil	

Therefore, to be at our optimum weight and health and for our over-all physical well-being, eat a low-fat diet with no more than 25% of your total daily caloric intake derived from fats. By replacing dairy products high in saturated fat with saturated fat-free, trans-fatty acid free, and monounsaturated and polyunsaturated fat enriched low-fat ANUTRA® BRAND DAIRY ALTERNATIVES, you're off to a great start!

STEP #5
Eat more fruits, vegetables, and other plant-based proteins (5 or more servings per day).

Throughout history, man has relied on the healing properties of plants and herbs, fruits, vegetables, seeds, nuts, and grains for food and medicine. Unfortunately, the demands of a fast-food, fast-paced world have changed much of that. More and more scientists and physicians are now turning back to nature to find solutions for modern diseases knowing that the key to our good health is so easily found in nature whether it be for food or medicines.

The findings are too numerous to ignore. Eating more fruits and vegetables and other plant-based proteins like ANUTRA® BRAND DAIRY ALTERNATIVES will help prevent a disease process that leads to heart attack and strokes as well as cancer. Fruits and vegetables provide the body with naturally occurring antioxidants that inhibit the oxidation of lipids that, when oxidized, ultimately leads to atherosclerosis. The process of atherosclerosis clogs blood vessels, which inhibits blood flow and causes heart attacks or strokes.

Let's also not forget the important compound we are going to learn more and more about throughout this century - phytonutrients. Fruits and vegetables are naturally abundant in these preventative and healing compounds. While more than 4,000 phytonutrients have been identified, fewer than 200 of them have been studied extensively.

I can't go through every fruit and vegetable and tell you which phytonutrients are found in each of them. It would take too long. But I will tell you what phytonutrients are found in the more common ones.

It is true that an apple a day may keep the doctor a away. Apples contain a variety of antioxidant phytonutrients that decrease LDL ("bad" cholesterol) oxidation. We already know that this is the type of cholesterol that builds up in our arteries and can lead to heart attacks and strokes. Studies have also proven that people who eat five or more apples per week have better lung function and a lower risk of asthma and other respiratory diseases. The pectin found in apples has also been shown to alleviate heartburn and chronic esophageal acid reflux disease.

Carotenoids, another powerful phytonutrient, are found in orange vegetables such as carrots, sweet potatoes, and squash, as well as in some dark green vegetables like broccoli and spinach. Women who eat carotenoid-enriched foods significantly reduce their risk of breast cancer. Isothiocyanates are the phytonutrients found in cruciferous vegetables. This nutrient helps the body produce enzymes that destroy cancer-causing compounds. Cruciferous vegetables include broccoli, brussel sprouts, cabbage, cauliflower, collard greens, and turnips. Men who eat more than two cups of cruciferous vegetables per week may reduce their risk of prostate cancer by 40%.

Berries are also very good for us. Cranberries and blueberries are very high in antioxidants. Studies show that they may have powerful anti-aging effects and help improve memory, balance, and coordination. The phytonutrients found in strawberries and red and black raspberries may inhibit the growth of colon and esophageal cancer cells.

I strongly suggest that you choose organic fruits and vegetables for they have fewer pesticide residues than non-organic produce. They have lower levels of pesticides, and they have much less overall pesticide toxicity than fruits and vegetables grown with chemicals, thereby reducing our consumption of xenobiotics such as estrogens that have been linked to breast, prostate, and testicular cancer. Also, the nutritional content of organically grown fruits and vegetables is higher than non-organic foods. Research confirms that, on average, organic produce contains significantly higher levels of vitamin C, iron, magnesium, and phosphorus providing us with what may be the difference between reaching the recommended daily allowances or not.

The bottom line is that there is an abundance of research on the health benefits of eating five to nine servings of fruits and vegetables per day. Incorporating the "5-9 a day" plan into your diet will have a profound effect on how you look and feel.

On the next three pages is a comprehensive list of fruits and vegetables which provides calories and nutritional information.

Table 1. Comparison of values in the USDA ORAC database per µmol TE/100g and µmol TE/typical serving

ORAC Database Foods ranked per 100g basis	µmol TE/100g
Spices, cloves, ground	314446
Spices, cinnamon, ground	267536
Spices, oregano, dried	200129
Spices, turmeric, ground	159277
Cocoa, dry powder, unsweetened	80933
Spices, cumin seed	76800
Spices, parsley, dried	74349
Spices, basil, dried	67553
Baking chocolate, unsweetened	49926
Spices, curry powder	48504
Chocolate, dutched powder	40200
Sage, fresh	32004
Spices, mustard seed, yellow	29257
Spices, ginger, ground	28811
Spices, pepper, black	27618
Thyme, fresh	27426
Marjoram, fresh	27297
Spices, chili powder	23636
Candies, chocolate, dark	20823
Candies, semisweet chocolate	18053

Table 1. Comparison of values in the USDA ORAC database per µmol TE/100g and µmol TE/typical serving

ORAC Database Foods ranked per typical serving		µmol TE/100g
Baking chocolate, unsweetened	1 square (29)	14479
Elderberries, raw	1/2 cup (72.5)	10655
Apples, Red Delicious, raw. with skin	1 med (182)	7781
Apples, Granny Smith, raw, with skin	1 med (182)	7094
Juice, Pomegranate, 100%	1 cup (253)	5923
Candies, chocolate, dark	1 oz (28.35)	5903
Plums, dried (prunes), uncooked	1/2 cup (87)	5700
Alcoholic beverage, wine, table, red	5 fl oz. (147)	5693
Artichokes, boiled	1/2 med (60)	5650
Apples, raw, with skin	1 med (182)	5609
Cranberries, raw	1/2 cup (55)	5271
Pears, raw	1 med (178)	5235
Prune juice, canned	1 cup (256)	5212
Apples, Gala, raw, with skin	1 med (182)	5147
Candies, semisweet chocolate	1 oz (28.35)	5118
Nuts, pecans	1 oz (28.35)	5086
Plums, black diamond, with peel, raw	1 fruit (66)	5003
Apples, Golden Delicious, raw, with skin	1 med (182)	4859
Blueberries, raw	1/2 cup (74)	4848
Apples, Red Delicious, raw, without skin	1 med (161)	4727

Fruit or Vegetable	5-A-Day Serving Size	Weight grams	Calories	Fiber grams	Vitamin.A IU	Vitamin.C mg	Potassium mg	Folate mcg
Apples	1 medium apple	138	81	4	35	8	159	4
Apple juice	3/4 cup juice	186	87	0	2	2	37	0
Apple juice (with added vitamin C)	3/4 cup juice	186	87	0	2	60	221	0
Apricots fresh	2 medium apricots	70	34	2	915	7	207	6
Apricots dried	4 dried apricot halves	14	33	1	1012	0	192	1
Artichokes, cooked	1 medium artichoke	120	60	6	110	12	425	61
Asparagus, cooked	6 medium spears or 1/2 cup chopped	72	22	1	245	10	144	131
Avocado, California	1/2 medium avocado	100	162	5	307	8	602	62
Bananas	1 medium banana	118	109	3	45	11	467	23
Beets, cooked	1/2 cup sliced beets	85	37	2	15	3	259	68
Beet Greens, cooked	1/2 cup greens	72	19	2	1835	18	655	10
Bell Peppers, sweet, green	1/2 cup chopped pieces	75	20	1	90	138	159	20
Bell Peppers, sweet, red	1/2 cup chopped pieces	75	20	1	2125	142	132	16
Bell Peppers, sweet, yellow	1/2 cup chopped pieces	75	20	1	235	66	131	16
Blackberries, fresh	1/2 cup	72	37	4	119	15	141	25
Blueberries, fresh	1/2 cup	72	41	2	35	9	65	0
Broccoli, raw	1/2 cup, cut pieces	44	12	1	340	41	143	31
Broccoli, cooked	1/2 cup, (about 2 spears)	78	22	2	540	58	228	39
Brussels Sprouts	1/2 cup, about 4 sprouts	78	30	2	280	48	247	47
Cabbage, Chinese, raw	1 cup shredded	70	9	1	2100	32	176	46
Cabbage, Chinese, cooked	1/2 cup	55	8	1	555	9	133	32
Cabbage, green, raw	1 cup shredded	70	18	2	45	23	172	30
Cabbage, green, cooked	1/2 cup	75	17	2	50	15	73	
Cabbage, red, raw	1 cup shredded	70	19	1	28	40	144	15
Cabbage, red, cooked	1/2 cup	75	17	2	20	26	105	10
Cantaloupe	1/2 cup, cubed pieces	80	28	1	2579	34	247	14
Carambola(a.k.a. star fruit)	1 medium carambola	91	42	3	310	27	207	18
Carrots, raw	1 medium carrot, raw	61	26	2	8580	6	197	9
Carrots, cooked	1/2 cup, sliced coins	78	35	3	9575	2	177	11
Carrots, baby, raw	8 medium carrots	80	30	2	12008	6	223	26
Cauliflower, raw	1/2 cup, cut pieces	50	13	1	5	23	152	29
Cauliflower, cooked	1/2 cup, cut pieces	62	14	1	5	27	88	27
Celery, raw	2 medium stalks	80	13	1	50	6	230	22
Chayote, raw	1/2 cup,chopped pieces	80	17	2	20	6	138	14
Cherries	1/2 cup, about 10 cherries	73	52	2	75	5	162	3
Clementine mandarin oranges	1 medium clementine	84	37	2	773	26	132	17
Collard Greens, cooked	1/2 cup, chopped	95	25	3	2973	17	247	88
Corn, cooked1/2 cup	82	89	2	90	5	204	38	
Cranberries, raw	1/2 cup	48	23	2	22	6	34	4
Cranberries, dried, unsweetened	1/4 cup	30	97	1	0	0	0	0
Cucumber1/2 cup, sliced	52	7	0.5	105	3	75	7	
Dates, dried	5 dates	42	114	3	10	0	271	5
Eggplant, cooked	1/2 cup, cubes	50	14	1	12	1	123	7
Field greens, assorted	1 cup	57	10	1	3000	5	-	-
Figs, raw	3 medium figs	150	111	5	105	3	348	9
Figs, dried	3 figs	57	144	5	75	1	405	5
Fruit cup, fresh or canned, in fruit juice	1/2 cup solids and juice	125	62	1	746	4	144	3

Fruit or Vegetable	5-A-Day Serving Size	Weight grams	Calories	Fiber grams	Vitamin.A IU	Vitamin.C mg	Potassium mg	Folate mcg
Grape juice, purple, unsweetened	3/4 cup juice	190	116	0	15	0	250	5
Grapefruit, pink or red	1/2 medium grapefruit	123	37	-	318	47	159	15
Grapefruit, white	1/2 medium grapefruit	118	39	1	12	40	175	12
Grapefruit juice, pink or red, unsweetened	3/4 cup	186	72	0	815	70	300	19
Grapefruit juice, white, unsweetened	3/4 cup	186	72	0	18	72	300	18
Grapes	1/2 cup, about 18 grapes	80	57	1	30	9	148	3
Green Beans, raw	1/2 cup, cut	55	17	2	367	9	115	20
Green beans, cooked	1/2cup, cut	62	21	2	416	6	187	20
Green peas, cooked	1/2 cup	80	62	4	534	8	134	47
Honeydew melon	1/2 cup, cubed pieces	85	30	0.5	34	21	230	5
Jicama	1/2 cup slices	60	23	3	5	12	90	7
Kiwifruit	1 large fruit	91	56	3	80	89	302	35
Lemons	1 medium lemon	84	22	5	15	83	157	-
Lettuce, iceberg	1 cup, shredded	56	7	1	182	2	87	31
Lettuce, green Leaf	1 cup, shredded	56	10	1	530	10	148	28
Lettuce, Romaine	1 cup, shredded	56	8	1	730	13	162	76
Mandarin oranges, canned	1/2 cup	125	46	1	1060	42	165	6
Mangos	1/2 medium mango	104	67	2	2015	29	161	14
Mushrooms, raw	1/2 cup, chopped	35	9	0.5	0	1	130	4
Nectarines	1 medium nectarine	136	67	2	505	7	288	5
Olives	1/3 cup, about 10 large olives	44	51	1	90	0	4	0
Oranges	1 medium orange	131	62	3	140	70	237	40
Orange juice (from concentrate)	3/4 cup juice	186	82	0.5	120	72	354	82
Orange juice (fresh)	3/4 cup juice	186	84	0.5	310	78	372	55
Papayas	1/2 cup cubed pieces (about 1/4 medium melon)	76	30	2	110	47	196	29
Peaches	1 medium peach	98	42	2	265	6	193	3
Pears	1 medium pear	166	98	4	15	7	208	12
Persimmons	1/2 medium persimmon	84	59	3	910	6	135	6
Pineapple, fresh	1/2 cup, chopped	78	38	1	10	12	89	8
Pineapple, canned, in its own juices	1/2 cup, solids and juice	125	75	1	47	0	151	6
Pineapple juice	3/4 cup juice	186	105	0.5	10	20	252	43
Pineapple juice with added vitamin C	3/4 cup juice	186	105	0.5	10	60	252	43
Plantain, cooked	1/2 cup slices	77	79	2	700	8	358	20
Plums	1 medium plum	66	36	1	105	6	114	1
Plums, dried (prunes)	1/4 cup, about 5 medium prunes	42	80	3	835	2	313	2
Pomegranates	1 medium pomegranate	154	105	1	0	9	399	9
Potatoes, no skin	1/2 cup, cooked/baked	61	57	1	0	8	239	6
Potatoes, with skin	1/2 small baked	67	75	2	0	9	288	8
Prune juice	3/4 cup juice	192	136	2	6	8	528	0
Pumpkin, canned	1/2 cup	123	42	4	27018	5	252	15

Fruit or Vegetable	5-A-Day Serving Size	Weight grams	Calories	Fiber grams	Vitamin.A IU	Vitamin.C mg	Potassium mg	Folate mcg
Raisins	1/4 cup	41	124	2	3	1	309	1
Radishes	1/2 cup raw, about 13 medium radishes	58	12	1	5	13	135	16
Raspberries	1/2 cup	62	30	4	40	15	93	16
Rhubarb, raw	1/2 cup	70	25	2	205	18	236	15
Rhubarb, cooked	1/2 cup	85	33	2	240	16	277	13
Spinach, raw	1 cup packed leaves	30	7	1	1010	8	167	58
Spinach, cooked	1/2 cup	90	21	2	3685	9	419	131
Squash, acorn, baked	1/2 cup	102	57	5	439	11	448	19
Squash, butternut, baked	1/2 cup	102	41	2	7151	15	291	19
Squash, zucchini, cooked	1/2 cup, slices	90	18	1	130	5	173	18
Strawberries	1/2 cup sliced berries, about 7 medium berries	83	25	2	22	46	138	15
Sweet Potatoes, baked	1/2 cup	100	103	3	21822	25	348	23
Swiss chard, cooked	1/2 cup	88	17	2	2747	16	480	8
Tangerines	1 medium tangerine	84	37	2	773	26	132	17
Tomatoes	1 medium tomato	123	26	1	380	23	273	18
Watermelon	1/2 cup, cubes	76	24	0	140	7	88	2

*Source: Dole5aday.com

STEP #6

Exercise at least 20 minutes every day! It can make a big difference in your mental alertness, physical appearance, and your overall health and well-being.

What is one of the easiest ways to lose weight; increase your stamina; build and maintain healthy bones, muscles and joints; prevent disease; and improve your mental alertness? Exercise, of course! Even a moderate amount of exercise can improve your health in many ways. It is a fact that when proper nutrition and physical activity are combined, they are the best foundation for a healthy lifestyle.

Yet why is it that something so simple, that is so good for us, and which takes so little time, is done by so few of us. The U.S. Department of Health and Human Services gives us these recent alarming statistics: nearly half of American youths aged 12-21 are not vigorously active on a regular basis; only 19% of all high school students are physically active for 20 minutes or more, five days a week; more than 60% of U.S. adults do not exercise regularly; and, approximately 25% of U.S. adults are not active at all. Exercise, one of the simplest and easiest keys to good health, is unused by so many!

I believe the industrial revolution played a major role in our becoming less active. Before automobiles, people walked and rode bicycles. Now, we drive our car even if we are going just a few blocks. The invention of the television didn't help either and turned many of us into "couch potatoes." Now, with the advent of the world-wide web, our activity level is even less.

Many of us have the preconceived notion that in order for exercise to be beneficial, it has to be strenuous and that we must become winded and sweat profusely. That is simply not true. Swimming, walking, bicycling - these, among many other activities, are good, safe, moderate exercises which most of us can do without much physical strain. Even greater health benefits can be derived from vigorous exercise. However, *excessively* vigorous exercise several times per week can sometimes cause injury, bone weakening, and menstrual abnormalities. So, while vigorous exercise is very good for us, even moderate physical activity, such as brisk walking for 20-30 minutes, done four or five days per week, can improve our health in many ways. Moderate exercise can:

Reduce the risk of premature death

Reduce the risk of heart disease

Reduce the risk of developing Type II diabetes

Reduce the risk of developing high blood pressure

Help reduce high blood pressure

Reduce the risk of developing colon cancer

Help control weight
(you can burn 7 to 10 calories per minute with certain activities)

Help build and maintain healthy bones, muscles, and joints

Reduce feelings of depression and anxiety

Promote psychological well-being

Here's how exercise may affect specific health issues:

BREAST CANCER

Several studies have proven that regular exercise may reduce the production of estrogen, which may accelerate cancer cells by the ovaries and by fat cells, and such a reduction in estrogen production may also lower the risk of breast cancer. It is also believed that women who exercise regularly usually have reduced body fat, which also may have protective breast cancer effects.

COLON CANCER

Many observational studies from around the world have proved that exercise may reduce colon cancer risk by up to 50%. It's not clear why being active inhibits colon cancer, but it could lower insulin production that has been linked to the disease. It may also lower levels of prostaglandins, small fatty molecules, that accelerate colon cell multiplication. Dr. Graham Colditz of Harvard University has been quoted as saying, "if every adult American increased their activity by walking the equivalent of half an hour a day, we would ... predict a 17% reduction in the risk of colon cancer." Based on this percent reduction, 18,000 lives would be saved each year.

MENTAL SHARPNESS

Exercise may help preserve your mental sharpness as you age. A recent study of approximately 6,000 women 65 years and older, without cognitive impairment or physical limitations, showed the least amount of cognitive decline over eight years. This occurred in those who exercised the most (walking 18 miles per week), while decline was greatest in those who exercised the least (walking half a mile per week). Decline decreased with each added mile.

BRAIN CELLS

There was a long-held belief in the field of neuroscience that we do not generate any new brain cells after birth. Recent tests on adult mice conducted at the Salk Institute in La Jolla, California proved just the opposite. Every time they exercised on running wheels, the adult mice doubled their number of new cells in the hippocampus, a brain area involved in memory and learning. It's not yet known whether the same thing happens with humans, but there's a strong chance that it does.

DEPRESSION

Research on physical activity and depression goes back to the 19th century. In recent decades, many studies have documented the benefits of exercise on mood in healthy and clinically depressed individuals. In the clinically depressed, studies overwhelmingly conclude that a moderate exercise program is an effective treatment and continued exercise inhibits the depression from returning. For anyone who exercises regularly, it may enhance our sense of mastery, divert our attention from areas of worry, concern, and guilt, and improve our health, physique, flexibility, and weight. Studies also suggest that exercise releases mood-altering hormones known as endorphins. Researchers continue to study the effects of exercise on the neurochemistry of mood regulation.

ENLARGED PROSTATE

Harvard Men's Health Watch reported an important finding suggesting that physical activity can reduce benign prostatic hyperplasia, or an enlarged prostate. The study showed a 25% lower risk of non-cancerous prostate enlargement in men who walked two to three hours a week than in men who seldom walked.

DIABETES

Many studies show that regular physical activity helps prevent or control diabetes. Exercise can lower your blood sugar level, helping to eliminate the need for insulin. It decreases your appetite and helps your own insulin work better. It also burns calories and leads to a reduction in body fat. Diets high in fat contribute to Type II diabetes by hindering the body's ability to process insulin.

BONES

Exercise is very important in the prevention and treatment of osteoporosis. It can slow mineral loss, help posture and balance, build muscle, strengthen bones, and improve overall fitness to reduce the risk of falls that may result in fractures. Just as your muscles can atrophy from lack of use, your bones can lose mass or density when no physical demands are placed on them.

Weight-bearing exercise, when muscles and bones go against gravity, and resistance exercises, which use muscular strength to improve muscle mass and strengthen bones, are equally important for building and maintaining healthy bones. Both types place physical demands on bones making them stronger and improving density.

ARTHRITIS

Both aerobic exercise and strength training, in moderation, can reduce joint swelling and pain as well as extend mobility.

THE HEART

People who exercise are less likely to develop heart problems due to stress, and people who are inactive are at greater risk for heart disease. This is an undisputed fact. Researchers also have evidence that exercise not only prevents heart disease, but also increases the odds of surviving a heart attack and preventing a second one.

Regular exercise lowers the risk of heart disease by boosting arterial blood oxygen supply, strengthening the heart muscle, lowering blood pressure, raising high-density lipoprotein (HDL) levels ("good" cholesterol), lowering low-density lipoprotein (LDL) levels ("bad" cholesterol), improving circulation, and increasing the heart's working capacity.

HIGH BLOOD PRESSURE

Approximately 60 million Americans have hypertension, or high blood pressure. This places them at a much greater risk of heart disease and stroke. Studies show that moderate exercise, when done on a regular basis, may lower both systolic (pressure during cardiac contractions - the "upper" line) and diastolic (pressure between cardiac contractions - the "lower" line) pressures by 5 to 10 points. It is believed that since exercise can reduce weight and body fat, reduce stress levels, and help widen constricted blood vessels to promote better circulation, it is beneficial in reducing high blood pressure.

OBESITY

Regular exercise and proper nutrition are the best ways to fight obesity. Exercise helps reduce body fat by building and strengthening muscle mass and increasing caloric metabolism. Exercise can also safeguard against other health risks associated with obesity such as Type II and adult-onset diabetes. A regular exercise program increases stamina, strength and mobility, improves self-image, and raises self-esteem.

BACK PAIN

Exercises that improve flexibility, strength, and endurance of the abdominal, back, and leg muscles will help prevent and alleviate back pain.

MORE...

Studies also point to the power of exercise to help prevent or control sleep disorders, gallstones, diverticular disease (an intestinal disorder) and more.

In summation, I believe exercise is the closest anti-aging device we have. There is no medicine or food that can hold as much promise for good health as a lifetime of physical exercise. It strengthens the heart and lungs, reduces body fat, increases circulation, relieves stress, keeps bones strong, and lowers blood pressure. Exercise strengthens and tones your muscles and increases flexibility. It increases your energy level, aids digestion, helps you sleep better, helps you look better, and improves self-esteem and self-confidence. You don't have to be a long-distance runner to accomplish this and remember, it's never too late to start!

A few simple and important exercise and dietary facts to remember...

- Fats have 9 calories per gram. All carbohydrates (simple and complex sugars) have 4 calories per gram. All proteins have 4 calories per gram, and alcohol has 7 calories per gram.

- Exercise can burn approximately 7-10 calories on average per minute.

- The average adult female needs about 1,500 calories per day.

- The average adult male needs about 2,000 calories per day.

- It's easy to figure out how many calories you need each day to maintain your weight, or lose or gain weight. Simply count the calories in each of your meals and reduce or add calories as needed.

- Please remember to compensate your caloric intake for exercising. If you are exercising and therefore burning calories, you can add additional calories each day to maintain your perfect weight.

- Be sure to eat at least 3 meals each day, or better yet, 5 to 6 small meals each day. It is best not to eat after 7:00 p.m. since we are typically less active after that time and burn less calories.

- If you are hungry in between meals or late at night, try drinking one of your favorite no or low calorie beverages such as water or tea. This can prevent you from snacking which can add additional calories you may not need.

- Develop a simple routine of aerobic exercise that you like such as walking, biking, swimming, jogging, tennis, or the like, and combine it with an anaerobic exercise such as sit-ups, pull-ups, push-ups, or whatever else you may enjoy doing.

- You don't need to go to the gym or buy expensive equipment to stay in great shape. Just think of our physically fit military. They don't use fancy gym equipment. They train without any frills and so can you.

STEP #7

Keep a positive attitude.
Be a good person.
Small changes will make a wonderful
difference in your life
and the world we live in.

Optimum health can only be achieved by having our mind, body, and spirit at their highest levels. A good spirit is usually found in *good* people and is more easily attained when our mind and body are in check. In the previous ANUTRASIZING™ steps, we discussed taking care of our physical health. We learned about why we should cut back on animal fat (saturated fats), eat more foods from the plant kingdom, and the importance of exercising. In ANUTRASIZING™ step seven, I will discuss how I believe our attitude can affect our health and how to reduce the stress in our lives.

Our attitude shapes how we deal with our emotions as it relates to other people and situations. It can be the best or the worst weapon we have, depending on how we use it, to help achieve optimum health. We now have very compelling evidence that mental attitudes are at the root of health and disease issues. Stressful lifestyles have been proven to exacerbate diseases while negative thoughts, moods, and feelings can have a significant effect on the onset of some diseases. On the other hand, positive attitudes and relaxed lifestyles seem to contribute to overall wellness.

I recently read an interesting excerpt from a radio interview with a noted sociologist. The sociologist said that with the use of satellites, television, and computers, we receive more information in one day than our ancestors received in a thousand days. Our brains, he said, have to process as much input in twenty-four hours as our brains used to process in twenty-four thousand hours resulting in major overload. I believe this to be true. No wonder we have more stress! He also said that 75% of all visits to primary care physicians are for stress-related disorders. I am not sure if that is factual, but I'll bet it's very close to that percentage.

The problem that most of us have is that we can be very self-defeating about many things that are both tangible and intangible. Self-defeating, negative emotions can have an adverse effect on longevity and learning to manage these feelings is important to leading a longer, healthier life. When we are happy and hopeful, we feel better. We feel very little stress and our bodies thrive under these conditions. When we are sad and feel despair, we feel badly. When these stressful emotions come to pass, we become predisposed to illness. There are many ways we can obtain a happy and hopeful feeling and become less prone to illness. It all stems from our attitude over which we have control.

Developing a healthy attitude comes from how your mind reacts to the stress in your life. Your attitude will be positive when you choose to take control of your emotions, passions, and moods. Of course, life without emotion and passion would be abnormal, but it's learning to control angry, impulsive tendencies and incorrect, negative responses that is the key. If we think carefully before responding and exercise self-control and reason, we will react much more positively to an unpleasant situation. Anger in this world is getting worse all the time. We should make every effort to realize we can not control the things people do or say which may make us angry. It is much healthier for us to stay in control of our negative emotions by not reacting, but by acting from positive emotions. To some of us, learning to control our negative emotions may come with just a little practice. To others, it may take some more time.

In ANUTRASIZING™ step six, I briefly discussed the importance of exercise and its role in reducing stress. It is probably the best and easiest stress-buster we know. When we exercise, our bodies produce substances known as endorphins. Endorphins naturally relieve pain and give us feelings of well-being and relaxation. They have a similar chemical structure to morphine. And we all know that when we are relaxed and feeling well, we have better control over our attitude/mind. Exercise also helps us fall asleep faster and helps reduce blood pressure. When we don't get enough sleep, we become irritable and anxious. When we are irritable and anxious, we put our bodies in a potentially dangerous mode to exacerbate illness. The same can be said for those with high blood pressure. They also can become irritable and anxious more easily than most. As I discussed in ANUTRASIZING™ step six, exercise is a great way to improve our mood, reduce blood-pressure, and help our overall well-being.

Another great way of achieving more control over our attitude/mind is through meditation. Therapists and other health professionals are discovering the various health benefits of meditation and recommending it to their patients. The state of relaxation that we can attain from meditating is also a tremendous stress-buster. There have been many scientific studies proving that meditation releases stress and in fact produces a reaction that is the exact opposite of stress; that is, a state of relaxation. It helps us to focus better, make conscious choices rather than reacting without thinking, opens our intuition, and helps us enjoy the life we are living. Meditation is not a religious practice, but is a personal and spiritual experience that most everyone can easily learn.

Yoga is another great way to manage and reduce our stress. There are several yoga techniques that can be used to alleviate stress and rejuvenate our mind, body, and spirit. Just taking ten to fifteen minutes a day to practice some of these simple techniques can be very refreshing to us. When we are stressed, our breathing becomes shallow and fast. This type of breathing reduces the amount of oxygen needed for general good health and causes an imbalance in our emotional and mental state. When we reach this state, our muscles tense and we become irritable and anxious. Yoga breathing techniques can make us more relaxed, and yoga stretches and postures can alleviate the physical effects of stress and tension.

So, if you want to start being more positive and reduce your stress, you need to develop good eating habits, exercise, meditate, and maybe even do some yoga. But first, you should start by smiling. When we smile, as the old song says, the whole world smiles with you. Wouldn't you rather see a smile than a scowl any day? And, when you see someone smiling, doesn't that relax you and make you feel better? When we are relaxed and happy there is less chance of our becoming ill or contracting a disease. Negative emotions, stress, and anxiety can affect our entire being. However, we can learn to manage our negative emotions by allowing ourselves a bit more time to think about the situation that is causing the negative emotion and by not immediately reacting in an angry way.

I have been involved in many think tanks at which we explored the secrets of motivation. While everyone has different ideas of what motivates them, it seemed to always come down to wanting to be the best we can be mentally, physically, and spiritually. When we decide to take the positive path, life is exciting and filled with purpose; but, if we become negative for whatever reason, and there is never a good reason, life will be filled with frustration and disappointments. Stay strong, stay positive, and remember, our quest for improved physical and mental health can all begin with just a smile and most important of all, always remember that God loves you in uncountable ways.

Part II

CONCLUSION

Now that you have read ANUTRA® "NATURE'S HEALTHIEST WHOLE FOOD", you may be trying to calculate my claim of how you will eliminate over 100,000 calories a year by turning to the ANUTRASIZING™ diet. It's really simple. You easily lose 68,000 of these calories when you incorporate ANUTRASIZING™ steps two and three into your daily nutrition. Including ANUTRASIZING™ step one and steps four through seven, will bring you an additional reduction of about 84,000 calories and will add tremendous value in your quest for a healthier and trimmer body and for a better world, both environmentally and economically.

According to the USDA, per capita cheese consumption in the United States is approximately 30 pounds. The good news regarding milk is that per capita milk consumption has been declining steadily. In 1985, Americans drank 26.2 gallons of milk per person, but by 1999, that number had declined to 23.5 gallons. It seems that the average consumer is starting to realize the harmful elements of drinking cow's milk, but they are not yet transferring that knowledge and understanding into their other dairy product choices.

I believe this is due to the effective advertising and marketing campaigns of cheese manufacturers and foodservice operators who present cheese as a wholesome food we cannot live without. In fact, they will tell us that the more cheese we eat, the better it is for us because of its calcium and vitamin benefits. What their advertising does not tell us about is the high saturated fat and cholesterol content of cheese, the dioxin levels, the dangerous IGF-1 hormone, and the fact that the body's absorption rate of calcium from cheese is not as high as its absorption rate from many vegetables.

Eating habits of certain cultures also enter into the steady increase in per capita cheese consumption. One of the major reasons that per capita cheese consumption is expected to rise over the next decade is because the rapidly increasing Hispanic population in the U.S. eats much more cheese than the average American consumer. Cheese consumption among Hispanic children is increasing the fastest among all ethnic groups in America and children of *all* ethnic backgrounds are the heaviest cheese consumers. Please think about this statistic. Which ethnic group has the highest rates of obesity and diabetes in America? The Hispanics do. Which age group has the fastest rising levels of obesity and diabetes in this country? The children of America do. Supersized portions, fast foods that include too much saturated fat (especially from dairy products), and less exercise are the primary contributors.

As I previously told you, when you follow steps two and three of THE ANUTRASIZING™ way of life, you can eliminate approximately 68,000 calories per year, or the equivalent of 17 pounds or more a year. The average American consumes about 83 pounds of fat each year. Approximately 20 pounds of this fat comes from dairy fat. If we switch to ANUTRA® BRAND DAIRY ALTERNATIVES, you will eliminate 65%, or 13 pounds of these 20 pounds of dairy fat. Since there are 4,000 calories to a pound of fat, eating ANUTRA® BRAND DAIRY ALTERNATIVES instead of conventional dairy products would reduce your annual dairy fat intake by a whopping 52,000 calories. That's 13 pounds! This is a simple and non-sacrificing way to not only eliminate a tremendous amount of calories, but also to get all the healthy benefits of rich phytonutrients in a much healthier product.

In addition to the 20 pounds of dairy fat consumed annually by the average American, we also consume about 8 pounds of hydrogenated vegetable fat per year. These hydrogenated fat oils come primarily from the margarine and shortening used to make cookies, donuts, crackers and many other common processed foods. By using Anutra® Butter instead of margarine and shortening, you would eliminate approximately 50%, or 4 of the 8 pounds of hydrogenated vegetable fat. The remaining 4 pounds of fat you would consume annually from Anutra® Butter is not harmful fat. It is unsaturated fat, with no trans-fatty acids, and contains only 3 grams per serving of mono- and poly-unsaturated fat - the healthy fats. Using the formula of 4,000 calories to a pound of fat would mean that replacing margarine and shortening with Anutra® Butter would eliminate another 16,000 calories, or 4 pounds per year! Anutra® Butter is the world's most nutritious butter and is the only one that contains high quality protein and other great nutritional benefits. Anutra® Butter is also lactose free.

Assuming we have incorporated the reduction in calories from using ANUTRA® BRAND DAIRY ALTERNATIVES into our eating habits, we would now have an annual intake of about 66 pounds of fat. We can reduce this by another 8 pounds per year by following ANUTRASIZING™ steps one and four. If we reduce our meat consumption by 10% weekly (step one) and, if we reduce our fat intake to 25% of our daily calories from fat (step four), we can further reduce our annual caloric intake by another 32,000 calories - the equivalent of 8 pounds!

All of us already know that exercise (ANUTRASIZING™ step six) is a known calorie reducer. I strongly recommend you follow this important step at least five times a week for at least twenty minutes each time. After dinner, instead of sitting down in front of the television, take a walk or go for a bike ride. If you can't go outdoors, walk in place or, if you have a staircase, go up and down it as many times as you are able. Create your own special twenty minutes of physical time that you will enjoy and don't forget to allow some time for peace and quiet.

Consider these times special in your life. They are yours, and yours alone, and only you control them. They are critical elements to your being the best that you can be. Daily exercise can reduce anywhere from 150-200 calories or more, depending on the type of activity we choose and the length of time we exercise. Most moderate exercises will burn an average of 7-10 calories every minute depending on the exercise. A bit more vigorous exercise done twenty minutes a day, five times a week, can burn as much as 1,000 calories per week. Everyone is different, so this number will vary, but potentially we can eliminate another 52,000 calories per year!

And last, but not least, being positive and smiling more (ANUTRA-SIZING™ step seven) makes us happier. When we are happy, we have a better self-image and we are more inclined to make the changes in our lives necessary to take the first six Anutrasizing™ steps. With a more positive and happier approach to life, we will be more likely to maintain the ANUTRASIZING™ stealth/health diet.

Now, let's add all these calorie reductions:

ANUTRA® BRAND DAIRY ALTERNATIVES		ELIMINATED CALORIES
Instead of conventional dairy	=	52,000
Anutra® Butter instead of margarine or shortening	=	16,000
Reducing meat consumption and 25% daily fat intake	=	32,000
Exercise - 20 minute/5 times per week (burn rate - 10 calories per minute)	=	52,000
TOTAL calories eliminated per year	=	**152,000**

152,000 calorie reduction = 38 less pounds!

If we consider that the 83 pounds of fat that we consume annually is approximately 332,000 calories from fat (4,000 calories equals one pound of fat), we can potentially reduce this amount to 232,000 fat calories, or 58 pounds of fat per year. My calculation does not include the fat calories eliminated by exercising. It includes only the dietary changes. This would be the equivalent of fasting approximately 50 days per year. Imagine that!

Last, but certainly not least, by eating more fruits, vegetables, and other plant-based proteins (ANUTRASIZING™ step five), we probably are replacing a higher calorie, high-fat snack, or a high-fat side dish to a main meal and will therefore automatically reduce our daily calories even further.

I believe it is also important to address in this conclusion an important macro event that is occurring and how this event will impact our personal future and the future of the world as we know it.

For most of the world's history, our population grew very slowly. It is estimated that the world population doubled every 1,000 years for the first eighteen centuries A.D. It took until approximately 1830 for the population to reach the billion mark, another one hundred years to reach the two billion mark, and, by 1960, the world population was three billion. Today, only a little more than forty years later, the world's population has reached 6.2 billion people and it is growing exponentially at an estimated annual rate of between 1.2% and 1.9% depending on which organizations' statistics you use. That's anywhere from 74 to 118 million more people every year! By the year 2050, the world population is expected to almost *double*.

About 95% of the population growth is expected to come from less developed countries and even more rapid growth will come from countries which are the least developed. However, the population of the world's *developed* countries is expected to stay about the same, and the populations of nearly forty of these developed countries are expected to decline substantially.

There are many problems associated with this projected massive population growth which will present a major challenge to the world. The most gripping problem is world hunger. The United Nations tell us that more than 800 million people are malnourished and malnutrition contributes to the death of 11,000 children each day. One starving child dies every eight seconds. In the last fifty years, almost 400 million people worldwide have died from hunger and poor sanitation. According to the USDA, in less developed countries, 91 out of every 1,000 children die before their fifth birthday. These facts are even more dramatic when you consider that even in the U.S., the wealthiest country in the world, 33 million people, including 13 million children, are hungry or are at risk of hunger. That's one in ten U.S. households, or 10% of the population!

The truth is that there is an abundance of nutritious food to feed the hungry. We are just not using these good foods for the right reasons. I am talking about healthy plant-based grains - ANUTRA®, soy, rice, oats, corn, wheat, barley, rye, millet, and more. As I told you in ANUTRASIZING™ step one, we are using 90% of the grain produced in the U.S., as well as high protein grain from third world countries, to feed livestock that will be slaughtered for its meat. We do this, as do all other meat producing countries, despite the fact that the process is wasting so much precious grain when there are so many in the world who are hungry. Remember, we get only one pound of meat for every 17 pounds of grain fed to livestock. And, when you consider that the wealthiest one-fifth of the world's people consume an unbelievable 86% of all goods and services and the poorest one-fifth consume 1%, we should realize that most of the meat produced throughout the world only feeds the relatively small amount of those who have the means to purchase it.

It is not just world hunger that will continue to be impacted by the tremendous burden of a doubled population in fifty years. Such a population boom, along with the world's growth centered economics, will continue to push the capacities of our ecosystems to their brink. I am talking about the basic life-support systems we take for granted - air, water, climate, the balance of nature - they are all being seriously threatened.

We are paying a huge environmental price for the steadily increasing demand on livestock farms to produce all types of meat and dairy products. There is a vicious cycle of soil erosion, salinization of soils, water pollution, and air pollution. There is the burning of our rainforest to make more land for grazing which causes another major environmental problem. The rainforests, which are vital to our existence for so many reasons, also serve as the world's thermostat. The hot and humid air generated by rainforests is carried away in rain clouds and then in air masses to eventually be distributed as rain and warmth over cooler climates. Oceanographers have confirmed that rapid and unpredictable shifts in climate are likely in as little as three to four decades. The continued burning of our rainforests will be a major reason for these climate shifts. There is also the problem of global warming, which is caused largely by burning fossil fuels, the release of methane gases by livestock into the atmosphere, and the release of carbon dioxide into the atmosphere when forests and grasslands (deforestation) are burned. These greenhouse gases are also contributing greatly to the climate changes around the world. Recently, a group of 2,500 climatologists told us that global warming, due to greenhouse gases, is unstoppable and will lead to 'widespread economic, social and environmental problems over the next century.' The U.S. is responsible for emitting about one-fifth of total global greenhouse gases. As I reported to you in ANUTRASIZING™ step one, livestock emit methane through belching and flatulation and are responsible for releasing approximately 60 million tons of methane into the atmosphere each year, representing 12% or more of the total methane released from all sources.

Life expectancy is another macro trend that is important for you to consider. Do you realize that Americans, who spend the most on healthcare in the world, rank a very disconcerting *forty-fourth in life expectancy* have more deaths from cancer and heart disease than any other country? After World War II, we ranked first in life expectancy. Our ranking is not expected to improve anytime soon, despite the fact that as a nation, we spend $1.7 trillion (17.3% of our GNP) annually on healthcare and overall healthcare spending is expected to more the double by 2010. If this does happen, how competitive is a nation that may potentially spend 35% of its GNP on healthcare?

The Japanese attained their number one life expectancy ranking because of their low rate of heart disease due to their traditional low-fat diet. It is, however, the consensus among health experts that the

Here are the latest life expectancy rankings of the top 50 countries according to the World Health Organization:

Healthy Life Expectancy Rankings
List by the CIA World Factbook (2007 estimates)

Rank	Member State	Total	Male	Female
		DALE in years		
1	Andorra	83.52	80.62	86.23
2	Macau (PRC)	82.27	79.44	85.25
3	Japan	82.02	78.67	85.56
4	San Marino	81.80	78.33	85.57
5	Singapore	81.80	79.21	84.59
6	Hong Kong (PRC)	81.68	78.99	84.60
7	Gibraltar (UK)	80.90	78.50	83.30
8	Sweden	80.63	78.39	83.00
9	Australia	80.62	77.80	83.59
10	Switzerland	80.62	77.75	83.63
11	France (Metropolitan)	80.59	77.35	84.00
12	Guernsey (UK)	80.53	77.53	83.64
13	Iceland	80.43	78.33	82.62
14	Canada	80.34	76.98	83.86
15	Cayman Islands (UK)	80.20	77.57	82.87
16	Italy	79.94	77.01	83.07
17	Monaco	79.82	75.99	83.85
18	Liechtenstein	79.81	76.24	83.40
19	Spain	79.78	76.46	83.32
19	Norway	79.78	76.46	83.32
19	Israel	79.78	76.46	83.32
22	Jersey (UK)	79.51	77.02	82.20
23	Faroe Islands (Denmark)	79.49	76.06	82.93
24	Greece	79.38	76.85	82.06
25	Austria	79.21	76.32	82.26
26	U.S. Virgin Islands (US)	79.20	75.40	83.22
27	Malta	79.15	76.95	81.47
28	Netherlands	79.11	76.52	81.82
29	Luxembourg	79.03	75.76	82.52
30	Montserrat (UK)	79.00	76.80	81.31
31	New Zealand	78.96	75.97	82.08
32	Germany	78.95	75.96	82.11
33	Belgium	78.92	75.75	82.24
34	Guam (US)	78.76	75.69	82.01
35	Saint Pierre & Miquelon (France)	78.76	76.41	81.23
36	United Kingdom	78.70	76.23	81.30
36	European Union	78.70	75.60	82.00
38	Finland	78.66	75.15	82.31
39	Isle of Man (UK)	78.64	75.30	82.17
40	Jordan	78.55	76.04	81.22
41	Puerto Rico (US)	78.54	74.60	82.67
42	Bosnia & Herzegovina	78.17	74.57	82.03
43	Bermuda (UK)	78.13	76.00	80.29
44	Saint Helena (UK)	78.09	75.19	81.15
45	United States	78.00	75.15	80.97
46	Cyprus	77.98	75.60	80.49
47	Denmark	77.96	75.65	80.41
48	Ireland	77.90	75.27	80.70
49	Portugal	77.87	74.60	81.36
50	Albania	77.60	74.95	80.53

Japanese will lose their number one ranking in the near future. It is expected that the negative health effects of a more "western" diet; that is eating high-fat foods such as red meat, along with higher lung cancer rates due to the dramatic post-World War II rise in smoking, will lower their ranking.

The U.S. ranking of forty-fourth may be shocking to us, but it shouldn't be if we think about it. As a nation, we still smoke a lot, we eat fast-foods that are typically high in saturated fats, more than half of Americans are either obese or overweight, most of us do not exercise regularly, we have more deaths from AIDS than most other advanced countries, and, our homicide rate, as compared to other advanced or industrial nations is fairly high.

In the U.S., those that typically eat a lot of meat and other high-fat foods are likely to be part of the 61% of Americans who are overweight and the more than 31% who are obese. These two conditions are the greatest precursors to heart disease, the number one cause of death; to cancer, the number two cause of death; and to diabetes, the dangerous disorder which is rising rapidly in this country. Being overweight has been linked to the incidence of approximately one-third of all cancer. Yet, according to the American Institute of Cancer Research, we are very slow to make the connection between our diet and cancer. I guess that is not surprising since we have known for many years of the health risks associated with a diet high in saturated fat, and yet unbelievably many of us still don't make the connection between our diets and coronary heart disease.

We need to start making serious changes TODAY. It has usually been up to our world leaders to initiate reforms that affect the macro events, but this time it is up to all of us. If we leave it to our world leaders, it may be too late. Never before has the individual had so much critical power to change the world for the better. These are SIMPLE lifestyle changes that we cannot afford not to make. Let's make the difference!

You can start by personally making these changes, by telling your family and friends to make these changes, by contacting your schools, colleges, hospitals, nursing homes, employee cafeterias, and any other facility that has a cafeteria and letting them know how important it is to ANUTRASIZE™. You can also write or call the following agencies:

- The American Dietetic Association
  1-800-877-1600; www.eatright.org;

- The American Heart Association
  1-800-242-8721; www.americanheart.org;

- The American Cancer Society
  1-800-ACS-2345; www.cancer.org;

- The American Diabetes Association
  1-800-342-2383; www.diabetes.org.

There are many other organizations that can help you get the message out. Tell your supermarket managers that you would like them to stock more products containing plant proteins and less animal fat products. I and my ANUTRA® associates will also be available to guide you in how to spread the ANUTRASIZING™ message. We can be reached at 1-888-532-3297 or through e-mail at: www.ANUTRA.COM. Let's do it now because it is the right thing to do for ourselves, our fellow man, and our world.

Part III

ANUTRASIZING™
RECIPES

SPECIAL NOTE ON ANUTRA® RECIPES

Each super nutritious and delicious recipe contains 5 grams of Anutra® with a minimum of 1,000 mg of Omega-3 370 ORAC Antioxidants, 1.5 grams of Fiber, and 425 mg of Lignans per serving

Simple way to AnutraSize™ *your favorite recipe*

Anutra® is so versatile that it easily works in just about any recipe. All you have to do to make your special recipe super-healthy is to add 5 grams of hydrated ground Anutra® per serving. Hydrating is easy, just add two parts water for each part Anutra®.

AnutraSize™

BREAKFAST

ANUTRASIZED™ ZUCCHINI BANANA BREAD WITH WALNUTS

Makes 10 Servings

1/2 cup Anutra® Butter
2 tablespoons 99% fat-free egg substitute or egg whites
1/2 banana - mashed
1 cup zucchini - skinned, shredded
1-1/4 teaspoon vanilla extract
1-1/2 cups all-purpose flour
1/2 cup sugar
1/2 teaspoon baking soda
1/2 teaspoon salt
1-1/2 teaspoons cinnamon
1/3 cup walnuts — chopped
4 tablespoons Anutra® Sour Cream
2/3 cup ANUTRA®
1-1/3 cup water

Preheat oven to 350 degrees. Mix first five ingredients (liquid/moist ingredients) in large bowl. Mix remaining dry ingredients. Add liquid/moist ingredients to dry mix. Mix well. Spray non-stick loaf pan, pour in batter and bake for 20 - 25 minutes. You may also place 1/3 cup of batter into a muffin pan (for individual portions) and bake for the same time.

Nutrition per serving: 256 Calories; 9g Fat (32% calories from fat); 6.5g Protein; 38.5g Carbohydrate; 0mg Cholesterol; 351mg Sodium. Exchanges: 1-1/2 Grain (Starch); 1/2 Lean Protein; 1 Fruit; 1 Fat; 1 Other Carbohydrate.

AUNT VIRGINIA'S APPLE CINNAMON ANUTRA® MUFFINS

Makes 10 Servings

1 cup diced apples
1-1/3 cup water
1/4 cup 99% fat-free egg substitute or egg whites
1/2 cup raisins
2 tablespoons canola oil
1 cup Anutra® Milk
1/3 cup all-purpose flour
1/2 teaspoon salt
1/4 cup sugar
1 tablespoon baking powder
1/2 teaspoon cinnamon
2/3 cup ANUTRA®

Heat oven to 400 degrees. Combine diced apples and 1 tablespoon of water and cook in microwave for 3 minutes. Combine eggs, apples, raisins, Anutra® Milk and remaining water, and oil. Using a wooden spoon, add mixture to dry ingredients. Lightly coat a non-stick muffin pan with vegetable spray. Place in preheated oven and bake for 20 minutes or until golden brown.

Nutrition per serving: 143 Calories;5.1g Fat (31% calories from fat); 3.1g Protein; 23.4g Carbohydrate; 0mg Cholesterol; 246mg Sodium. Exchanges: 1/2 Grain (Starch); 1 Fruit; 1/2 Fat; 1/2 Other Carbohydrate.

FRENCH TOAST ANUTRASIZED™

Makes 4 Servings

1/2 cup water
2 cups 99% fat-free egg substitute or egg whites
1/2 cup Anutra® Milk
1/4 cup Anutra® Cream Cheese
1/4 cup sugar
1/2 teaspoon cinnamon
1/4 cup ANUTRA®
1/4 loaf Italian bread — sliced 1/2-inch thick
vegetable cooking spray
2 tablespoons Anutra® Butter

Heat large non-stick skillet to medium temperature. In a large bowl, add first 7 ingredients. Combine and beat until fluffy. Take cut slices of bread and dip quickly in mix, covering both sides of the bread. Spray heated pan and place dipped breads approx 1 inch apart. Let cook approx 2-3 minutes. Flip and let cook again 2-3 minutes. Repeat process until toast is golden brown and firm. Serve immediately with Anutra® Butter on top.

Nutrition per serving: 262 Calories; 6.3g Fat (21% calories from fat); 17.1g Protein; 34.4g Carbohydrate; 0mg Cholesterol; 522mg Sodium. Exchanges: 1 Grain (Starch); 1-1/2 Lean Protein; 1 Fruit; 1/2 Fat; 1 Other Carbohydrate.

OVEN BAKED ONION AND ANUTRA® CHEESE FRITTATA

Makes 6 Servings

1 teaspoon olive oil
1-1/2 small onion — minced
1/2 cup Anutra® Parmesan Cheese
1 cup Anutra® Mozzarella Shreds
1/4 cup Anutra® Cream Cheese
2 cups 99% fat-free egg substitute or egg whites
3/4 teaspoon oregano
1-1/2 dashes nutmeg
salt and pepper — to taste
1/3 cup ANUTRA®
2/3 cup water

Heat oven to 350 degrees. Sauté onion in oil until golden. Beat eggs with Anutra® Cream Cheese until broken up and fluffy. Add all other ingredients into the pan. Mix well. Pour into a sprayed glass baking dish and bake for about 30 minutes, or until set and top is golden.

Add other favorites to this frittata: cooked potatoes, artichoke hearts, peppers, spinach, mixed summer vegetables and other Anutra® cheeses.

Nutrition per serving: 169 Calories; 6.9g Fat (31% calories from fat); 17.5g Protein; 9.6g Carbohydrate; 0mg Cholesterol; 594mg Sodium. Exchanges: 2-1/2 Lean Protein; 1/2 Vegetable; 1/2 Fat.

SILVER DOLLAR BANANA AND WALNUT ANUTRA® MILK PANCAKES

Makes 6 Servings

2 cups all-purpose flour
1/2 teaspoon salt
3 tablespoons sugar
3/4 teaspoon baking soda
1 tablespoon baking powder
1-1/2 cups Anutra® Milk
1/4 cup 99% fat-free egg substitute or egg whites
2 tablespoons Anutra® Butter
1 teaspoon vanilla extract
1-1/2 cups banana
1/2 cup walnuts
Aunt Jemima® Lite syrup (optional)
1/3 cup ANUTRA®
2/3 cup water

Combine flour, salt, sugar, baking soda and baking powder in a large mixing bowl. In a separate bowl, whisk together the Anutra® Milk, Anutra® Butter and eggs. Add bananas and walnuts. Add the wet ingredients to the dry. Stir with a wooden spoon to combine. (The batter will be slightly lumpy.) Spray a griddle or skillet lightly with cooking spray; heat until it is moderately hot. Drop the batter onto griddle, using a 2 oz. ladle, leaving about 1 inch of space between pancakes. Cook the pancakes until the undersides are brown, the edges begin to dry, and bubbles begin to break the surface of the batter, about 1 - 2 minutes. Turn the pancakes and cook them until the second side is brown. Repeat using the remaining batter. Serve immediately.

Top with Anutra® Butter and Aunt Jemima® Lite syrup.

Nutrition per serving: 366 Calories; 10.2g Fat (25% calories from fat); 11.8g Protein; 59.3g Carbohydrate; 0mg Cholesterol; 605mg Sodium. Exchanges: 2-1/2 Grain (Starch); 1/2 Lean Protein; 1-1/2 Fruit; 1/2 Other Carbohydrates.

SOUTHWEST CHEDDAR JALAPEÑO ANUTRASIZED™ SCRAMBLED EGGS

Makes 4 Servings

vegetable cooking spray
1/2 cup onion — cut in 1/4 inch pieces
2 cups 99% fat-free egg substitute or egg whites
1/4 cup Anutra® Cream Cheese
2 tablespoons Anutra® Milk
4 Anutra® Cheddar Jalapeño Slices — cut in 1/2 inch strips
1/4 cup ANUTRA®
1/2 cup water

In mixing bowl, beat eggs, Anutra® Cream Cheese, Anutra® Butter Anutra® Milk and water until fluffy; set aside. Heat medium sized non-stick skillet to medium high heat. Spray vegetable cooking spray, add onion to skillet and cook for approx 1 minute. Spray pan again and pour mixture into skillet with onions, add Anutra® Cheddar Jalapeño slices and scramble until eggs are dry.

Serve with plenty of fresh fruit and homemade Anutrasized™ muffins.

Nutrition per serving: 173 Calories; 6.6g Fat (34% calories from fat); 19.5g Protein; 9g Carbohydrate; 0mg Cholesterol; 675mg Sodium. Exchanges: 2 Lean Protein; 1/2 Vegetable; 1/2 Fat.

SPANISH ANUTRA® PEPPER JACK OMELET

Makes 1 Serving

OMELET
1/2 cup 99% fat-free egg substitute or egg whites
1 tablespoon Anutra® Cream Cheese
1 tablespoon Anutra® Milk
salt and pepper

SPANISH FILLING
vegetable cooking spray
1 clove garlic — minced
1 tablespoon chopped onions
1/2 stalk celery — chopped
1/4 teaspoon oregano
1 tablespoon chopped green bell pepper
1 teaspoon chopped olives — (optional)
1 tablespoon chopped parsley — (optional)
1 small tomato, chopped, peeled — drained
1 Anutra® Pepper Jack Slice — cut in half
1 tablespoon ANUTRA®
2 tablespoons water

Heat a non-stick cooking pan to medium high heat. Lightly cover with vegetable cooking spray and prepare filling first by sautéing the onions and garlic until clear and light golden; add parsley, celery, peppers, herbs and tomatoes. Add the olives last. Set aside. Prepare omelet: Beat all the omelet ingredients until fluffy. Lightly cover non-stick skillet with vegetable cooking spray, heat to medium and add the egg mixture. Using a small spatula, run around the edges of the skillet tipping the skillet so the uncooked egg from the center of the pan can run under the bottom of the cooked egg. Continue to do this until the egg in the center is still a little moist. Fill with Spanish mixture, place Anutra® Pepper Jack Cheese on top of mixture and fold one half of the omelet over. Serve or roll the omelet with three folds as you turn it onto the plate.

Nutrition per serving: 194 Calories; 6.6g Fat (31% calories from fat); 19.3g Protein; 16.1g Carbohydrate; 0mg Cholesterol; 609mg Sodium. Exchanges: 2 Lean Protein; 1-1/2 Vegetable; 1 Fat.

SPICED BREAKFAST ANUTRA® SOUFFLE

Makes 10 Servings

10 bread slices
3 tablespoons Anutra® Butter
vegetable cooking spray
1 cup Anutra® Cheddar Shreds
1 cup Anutra® Mozzarella Shreds
3 cups 99% fat-free egg substitute or egg whites
1/2 cup Anutra® Milk
1/4 cup Anutra® Cream Cheese
2/3 cup ANUTRA®
1-1/3 cup water
1 teaspoon minced onions
1/2 teaspoon curry powder
1/8 teaspoon cayenne pepper
1/4 teaspoon paprika
1 teaspoon Worcestershire sauce
1 teaspoon dry mustard
1 pinch saffron — optional

Spray the sides and bottom of 9" x 13" x 2" pan with vegetable cooking spray. Remove crusts from bread and butter the bread. Cut into cubes. Place half the bread in the pan and sprinkle with half the cheeses. Add rest of bread cubes and sprinkle with remaining cheeses. Combine beaten eggs, Anutra® Cream Cheese, Anutra® Milk, ANUTRA®, water, onion, curry powder, cayenne pepper, Worcestershire sauce, dry mustard, saffron and paprika. Pour over the bread and cheese. Cover tightly and refrigerate overnight or at least 8 hours. Bake in preheated 325 degree oven for 1 hour or until lightly browned and knife inserted in center comes out clean.

Prepared the night before, this dish makes a wonderful and quick breakfast — just pop it in the oven and serve.

Nutrition per serving: 202 Calories; 7.1g Fat (32% calories from fat); 15.4g Protein; 19g Carbohydrate; 0mg Cholesterol; 632mg Sodium. Exchanges: 1 Grain (Starch); 1-1/2 Lean Protein; 1/2 Fat.

ANUTRA® SPRING VEGETABLE EGG WHITE OMELET

Makes 1 Serving

3 egg whites
1 tablespoon ANUTRA®
salt and pepper to taste
2 tablespoons Anutra® Milk
2 tablespoons water
4 snow pea pods, fresh, whole — julienned
1/2 ounce red pepper — julienned
1/2 ounce yellow squash — julienned
1/2 ounce zucchini — julienned
1/2 ounce red onion — julienned
1/2 teaspoon cumin powder
1 Anutra® Pepper Jack Slice
vegetable cooking spray
2 tablespoons ANUTRA® CHEDDAR SAUCE (see recipe page 303)

Place eggs, Anutra®, water, and Anutra® Milk in a mixing bowl; whip until light and foamy. Coat omelet pan with cooking spray, sauté the vegetables over high heat. Season vegetables with salt, pepper and cumin; set aside. Coat the same pan with more cooking spray. Place the egg mixture in the pan. Cooking over high heat, make an omelet. Place the pepper jack and sautéed vegetables on the inside of the omelet. Fold the omelet over and place on a serving dish. Cover the omelet with Anutra® Cheddar Sauce.

Nutrition per serving: 199 Calories; 6.6g Fat (30% calories from fat); 22.5g Protein; 11.8g Carbohydrate; 0mg Cholesterol; 714mg Sodium. Exchanges: 3 Lean Protein; 1/2 Vegetable.

STEALTH ANUTRASIZED™ OATMEAL

Makes 1 Serving

1-1/4 cup Anutra® Milk
1/2 cup Quaker® oats, rolled (raw)
1/2 teaspoon vanilla
1 tablespoon honey
1 tablespoon ANUTRA®

Stove top: Boil Anutra® Milk. Stir in Oats. Cook about five minutes over medium heat.

Microwave: Combine Anutra® Milk, Anutra®, and oats in medium microwave bowl. Microwave on high 2-1/2 to 3 minutes; stir before serving.

We call this stealth because it not only provides 8 grams of soy protein, but the oatmeal is a great source of soluble fiber and is also linked to a decreased risk of heart disease.

Add cinnamon, apple, strawberries, granola or any other of your favorite toppings for variety.

Nutrition per serving: 364 Calories; 7.1g Fat (18% calories from fat); 16.5g Protein; 60.3g Carbohydrate; 0mg Cholesterol; 132mg Sodium. Exchanges: 3 Grain (Starch); 1 Lean Protein; 1/2 Fat; 1 Other Carbohydrate.

ANUTRA® MILK AND BUTTER PANCAKES

Makes 6 Servings

2 cups all-purpose flour
1/3 cup ANUTRA®
2/3 cups water
1/2 teaspoon salt
3 tablespoons sugar
3/4 teaspoon baking soda
1 tablespoon baking powder
1-1/2 cups Anutra® Milk
1/4 cup 99% fat-free egg substitute or egg whites
2 tablespoons Anutra® Butter
1 teaspoon vanilla extract
Aunt Jemima® Lite syrup (optional)

Combine flour, salt, sugar, baking soda, and baking powder in a large mixing bowl. In a separate bowl, whisk together the Anutra® Milk, water Anutra® Butter and eggs. Add the wet ingredients to the dry. Stir with a wooden spoon to combine. (The batter will be slightly lumpy.) Lightly spray a griddle or skillet with cooking spray; heat until it is moderately hot. Drop the batter onto griddle, using a 2 ounce ladle, leaving about 1 inch of space between pancakes. Cook the pancakes until the undersides are brown, the edges begin to dry, and bubbles begin to break the surface of the batter, about 1 - 2 minutes. Turn the pancakes and cook them until the second side is brown. Repeat using the remaining batter. Serve immediately with Anutra® Butter and Aunt Jemima® Lite syrup as a topping.

For variety, add walnuts, blueberries or top with fresh strawberries.

Nutrition per serving: 251 Calories; 4g Fat (14% calories from fat); 8.7g Protein; 44.9g Carbohydrate; 0mg Cholesterol; 604mg Sodium. Exchanges: 2-1/2 Grain (Starch); 1/2 Lean Protein; 1/2Fruit; 1/2 Other Carbohydrate.

ANUTRA® CHEDDAR GRITS

Makes 4 Servings

1/2 cup grits
1/4 cup ANUTRA®
2-1/2 cups water
1/4 cup 99% fat-free egg substitute or egg whites
1 cup Anutra® Cheddar Shreds
1 tablespoon Worcestershire sauce
1/4 cup Anutra® Butter
pinch cayenne pepper — to taste
1/4 cup bread crumbs
salt and pepper — to taste

Cook grits until thick. Beat eggs and Anutra® Butter until fluffy. Stir in cheese, Worcestershire sauce, and cayenne. Stir into grits. Spray 8" x 8" casserole dish, add grit mixture, sprinkle with bread crumbs, and bake at 350 degrees for 45 minutes.

Nutrition per serving: 236 Calories; 8.7g Fat (33% calories from fat); 11.8g Protein; 27.4g Carbohydrate; 0mg Cholesterol; 603mg Sodium. Exchanges: 1-1/2 Grain (Starch); 1 Lean Protein; 1/2 Fat.

ANUTRA® CHEDDAR HASH BROWNS

Makes 12 Servings

1/2 cup low sodium vegetable broth
3/4 cups ANUTRA®
1 cup water
2 cups Anutra® Cheddar Shreds
3/4 cup Anutra® Sour Cream
1/4 cup Anutra® Butter
1/4 cup onion — diced small
1/2 teaspoon garlic powder
1-1/4 pounds potatoes, shredded
vegetable cooking spray

Preheat oven to 350 degrees. Combine all ingredients except shredded potatoes. Mix until well blended. Fold in shredded potatoes. Add mixture to lightly coated 2 quart baking dish. Bake for 40-45 minutes.

Nutrition per serving: 104 Calories; 6.5g Fat (56% calories from fat); 6.4g Protein; 6g Carbohydrate; 0mg Cholesterol; 336mg Sodium. Exchanges: 1 Lean Protein; 1/2 Fat.

ANUTRA® CHEDDAR POTATO AND ONION OMELET

Makes 1 Serving

OMELET:
1/2 cup 99% fat-free egg substitute or egg whites
1 tablespoon ANUTRA®
1 tablespoon Anutra® Cream Cheese
1 tablespoon Anutra® Milk
2 tablespoons water
pinch salt and pepper
2 tablespoons Anutra® Cheddar Shreds
vegetable cooking spray

FILLING:
3 tablespoons onion — cut in 1/4" pieces
1/2 cup potatoes, shredded
1/4 teaspoon ground nutmeg

Heat non-stick skillet to medium high heat. Apply cooking spray and add onion and potatoes. Cook for 2 minutes. Take mixture out of pan and place on side. Mix and beat together all omelet ingredients until fluffy. Apply vegetable cooking spray to skillet heated to medium and add the egg mixture. Using a small spatula, run around the edges of the skillet, tipping the skillet so the uncooked egg from the center of the pan can run under the bottom of the cooked egg. Continue to do this until the egg in the center is still a little moist, add onion and potato mixture, sprinkle with nutmeg, add Anutra® Cheddar Shreds then fold one half of the omelet over. Serve.

Nutrition per serving: 153 Calories; 5.4g Fat (32% calories from fat); 17g Protein; 9.6g Carbohydrate; 0mg Cholesterol; 484mg Sodium. Exchanges: 2 Lean Protein; 1/2 Vegetable; 1/2 Fat.

ANUTRA® EGG WHITES A LA SWISS

Makes 6 Servings

2 tablespoons Anutra® Cream Cheese
2 cups 99% fat-free egg substitute or egg whites
1/3 cup ANUTRA®
2/3 cup water
4 Anutra® Swiss Slices
6 whole wheat english muffins — halved
3 tablespoons Anutra® Butter
1/2 cup minced green onions
1 teaspoon freshly grated nutmeg
2 tablespoons Anutra® Parmesan Cheese

In a small bowl, mix together Anutra® Cream Cheese Anutra®, water and eggs. In a large skillet over medium-high heat, spray pan with non-stick cooking spray and scramble egg mixture adding Anutra® Swiss Slices. Cook until eggs are firm and cheese has melted. Hold in warm oven or cover with foil. Toast english muffins and spread each half with 1/2 tablespoon of Anutra® Butter. Place a 1/2 cup of the scrambled egg whites on each half. Sprinkle each half with green onions, nutmeg, and Anutra® Parmesan Cheese. Serve immediately.

Nutrition per serving: 263 Calories; 7.1g Fat (24% calories from fat); 18.3g Protein; 33g Carbohydrate; 0mg Cholesterol; 745mg Sodium. Exchanges: 2 Grain (Starch); 1-1/2 Lean Protein; 1/2 Fat.

ANUTRA® EGGS BENEDICT

Makes 4 Servings

2 whole wheat english muffins — split in half
1-1/2 tablespoons Anutra® Butter
4 vegetarian canadian bacon slices
2 cups 99% fat-free egg substitute or egg whites
1/4 cup ANUTRA®
1/2 cup water
1/4 cup ANUTRA® CHEDDAR SAUCE (see recipe page 303)

Preheat oven to 350 degrees. Heat non-stick skillet and bring up to medium-high heat. Lightly coat with vegetable spray. Add egg substitute, Anutra® and water cook and set aside. Toast english muffin halves and warm vegetarian canadian bacon in oven for approx 2 minutes. Spread 1 teaspoon of Anutra® Butter on top of muffin. Place muffin half on serving plate and top with vegetarian bacon. Place 1/2 cup of eggs on top of the vegetarian bacon and pour 1 tablespoon of Anutra® Cheddar Sauce over entrée.

Nutrition per serving: 180 Calories; 4.8g Fat (24% calories from fat); 16.1g Protein; 18.8g Carbohydrate; 0mg Cholesterol; 509mg Sodium. Exchanges: 1 Grain (Starch); 1-1/2 Lean Protein; 1/2 Fat.

ANUTRA® MILK SMOOTHIE

Makes 1 Serving

1 cup Anutra® Milk
1 tablespoon ANUTRA®
1/2 cup frozen strawberries
1/3 cup frozen blueberries
1/2 cup frozen banana
1 teaspoon honey

Place all ingredients in blender. Blend until smooth. Serve.

The Anutra® Milk® Smoothie is an excellent meal replacement and good way to start the day.

Nutrition per serving: 387 Calories; 5.6g Fat (13% calories from fat); 12.1g Protein; 80.1g Carbohydrate; 0mg Cholesterol; 133mg Sodium. Exchanges: 1 Grain (Starch); 1 Lean Protein; 4 Fruit; 1/2 Other Carbohydrate.

ANUTRA® OMELET IN A PITA

Makes 4 Servings

1-1/2 cups 99% fat-free egg substitute or egg whites
1/4 cup Anutra®
1/2 cup water
1/4 cup Anutra® Cream Cheese
1/2 teaspoon dried whole basil
1/8 teaspoon salt
1/4 teaspoon hot pepper sauce
vegetable cooking spray
1 cup sliced fresh mushrooms
1/2 cup thinly sliced green onions
1/2 cup Anutra® Shreds — Monterey Jack and Cheddar Blend
2 pita bread pockets, cut in half — 6-inch
8 slices unpeeled tomato, 1 medium — 1/4-inch thick

Combine first 8 ingredients in a bowl; beat until fluffy, and set aside. Coat a non-stick skillet with cooking spray; place over medium heat until hot. Add mushrooms and green onions; sauté 2 minutes. Increase heat to medium-high, and add egg mixture; cook 2 minutes. Cover and cook an additional minute or until center is set. Remove from heat; top with cheese. To serve, slide omelet onto serving plate; cut into four portions. Line each pita half with 2 tomato slices; place one omelet portion into each half.

Nutrition per serving: 217 Calories; 5.6g Fat (23% calories from fat); 17.2g Protein; 25.4g Carbohydrate; 0mg Cholesterol; 673mg Sodium. Exchanges: 1 Grain (Starch); 1-1/2 Lean Protein; 1/2 Vegetable; 1/2 Fat.

ANUTRA® PEACH AND BERRY SMOOTHIE

Makes 2 Servings

1 cup frozen peach slices
1 cup Anutra® Milk
2 tablespoon ANUTRA®
2 teaspoons vanilla extract
1/2 cup raspberries
1 cup ice

Combine everything in a blender. Whirl until smooth.

Nutrition per serving: 229 Calories; 3.6g Fat (14% calories from fat); 6.6g Protein; 43.4g Carbohydrate; 0mg Cholesterol; 76mg Sodium; Exchanges: 1/2 Grain (Starch); 1/2 Lean Protein; 2 Fruit.

ANUTRA® PEPPER JACK BREAKFAST BURRITO

Makes 1 Serving

3/4 cup 99% fat-free egg substitute or egg whites — or egg whites
1 tablespoon ANUTRA®
1 flour tortilla
2 tablespoons fat-free refried beans
1/2 teaspoon fresh cilantro
1 pinch cumin
2 tablespoons Anutra® Shreds — Pepper Jack and Cheddar Blend
1 tablespoon salsa

Spray egg pan with cooking spray; place over medium high heat. Cook eggs and Anutra® until firm. Set aside. In bowl, mix refried beans, cilantro and cumin. Spread refried beans over top half of tortilla. Place eggs in the center of the tortilla. Place salsa over eggs, then Anutra® Shreds over salsa. Fold in the sides and roll (keeping the sides folded in). Place seam side down on a plate and microwave for 1 minute. Cut in half and serve.

Nutrition per serving: 271 Calories; 6.1g Fat (20% calories from fat); 22.6g protein; 30.3g Carbohydrate; 0mg Cholesterol; 766mg Sodium. Exchanges: 1-1/2 Grain (Starch); 2-1/2 Lean Protein; 1/2 Fat.

ANUTRA® PUMPKIN CRANBERRY LOAF

Makes 12 Servings

1-1/2 cups all-purpose flour
1/2 cup whole wheat flour
3/4 cup ANUTRA®
2/3 cup firmly packed dark brown sugar
1/2 cup sugar
2 teaspoons baking powder
1/4 teaspoon salt
1-3/4 teaspoons pumpkin pie spice
1 cup canned pumpkin
1/4 cup Anutra® Milk
1 cup water
1/4 cup Anutra® Butter
1/4 cup Anutra® Sour Cream
1-1/2 teaspoons vanilla extract
1/2 cup 99% fat-free egg substitute or egg whites — lightly beaten
3/4 cup coarsely chopped cranberries
vegetable cooking spray
1/4 cup chopped pecans

Combine the first 7 ingredients in a large bowl; make a well in center of mixture. Combine pumpkin, Anutra® Milk, water Anutra® Butter, Anutra® Sour Cream, and eggs; add to dry ingredients, stirring just until dry ingredients are moistened. Fold in cranberries. Pour batter into a 9" x 5" loaf pan coated with cooking spray; sprinkle pecans over batter. Bake at 350 degrees for 1 hour and 5 minutes or until a wooden pick inserted in center comes out clean. Let cool in pan 10 minutes on a wire rack; remove from pan, and let cool completely on wire rack.

Nutrition per serving: 202 Calories; 5.4g Fat (24% calories from fat); 5.2g Protein; 34.5g Carbohydrate; 0mg Cholesterol; 172mg Sodium. Exchanges: 1 Grain (Starch); 1/2 Vegetable; 1/2 Fruit; 1/2 Fat; 1 Other Carbohydrate.

ANUTRA® VEGETABLE FRITTATA

Makes 8 Servings

1/2 tablespoon olive oil
3/4 cup onion — cut in 1/2-inch cubes
3/4 cup green bell peppers — cut in 1/2-inch cubes
3/4 cup mushrooms — sliced 1/4-inch thick
3/4 cup canned tomatoes — drained
1 teaspoon oregano
1 teaspoon basil
1/2 teaspoon garlic powder
pinch salt and pepper
1 cup Anutra® Shreds — Monterey Jack and Cheddar Blend
2 tablespoons Anutra® Parmesan Cheese
1-1/2 cups 99% fat-free egg substitute or egg whites
1-1/2 cups potatoes, shredded
1/2 cup Anutra®

Preheat oven to 325 degrees. Using non-stick pan, heat to medium-high heat. Add olive oil. Add onion and mushrooms, sauté for 1 minute. Add seasonings, toss. Add peppers and tomatoes and cook for 3 minutes. Add potatoes and cook for 1 additional minute. Take pan off burner and toss in Anutra® Shreds and 1 tablespoon of Anutra® Parmesan. Add 1/4 cup Anutra® to eggs and stir than pour eggs into pan (do not stir) and cover with foil. Place in oven. Let bake for 12 minutes. Remove foil and let bake 10-15 more minutes until firm. Remove from oven and gently go around sides with a knife or spatula to loosen from pan. Gently slide out of pan onto serving plate. Sprinkle remaining Anutra® Parmesan on top and 1/4 cup Anutra®.

Nutrition per serving: 105 Calories; 4.7g Fat (40% calories from fat); 9g Protein; 7.4g Carbohydrate; 0mg Cholesterol; 338mg Sodium. Exchanges: 1 Lean Protein; 1/2 Vegetable.

ANUTRA® VEGETABLE QUICHE

Makes 6 Servings

3 egg roll wrappers
1/2 cup Anutra® Mozzarella Shreds
1 teaspoon olive oil
1/2 cup yellow squash — diced
1/2 cup zucchini — diced
1/4 cup onion — diced
1/4 teaspoon garlic — minced
1/2 teaspoon salt
1/4 teaspoon ground black pepper
2 tablespoons Anutra® Parmesan Cheese
1/3 cup ANUTRA®
1 cup Anutra® Milk
2/3 cup water
2 egg whites
vegetable cooking spray

Preheat oven to 350 degrees. Lightly spray a 12-compartment muffin tin with non-stick vegetable spray. Cut the egg roll skins into quarters. Press 3-1/4 pieces of egg roll skin into each muffin tin to form a shell. In a skillet, sauté the zucchini, yellow squash, and onion in the olive oil and garlic. Season with salt and pepper. Remove from heat. Spoon this mixture evenly among the 12 muffin compartments. Place 1 teaspoon of Anutra® Parmesan into each tin, followed by 1 tablespoon of Anutra® Mozzarella Shreds. In a mixing bowl, combine the Anutra® Milk Anutra®, water and eggs, mix together well. Pour the mixture over the vegetables and Anutra® Shreds until just covered. Bake in oven for approx 30 minutes or until quiches are set. Remove from oven and allow to cool for 15 minutes before removing from muffin tin.

Nutrition per serving: 103 Calories; 4.5g Fat (39% calories from fat); 7.4g Protein; 9g Carbohydrate; 0mg Cholesterol; 405mg Sodium. Exchanges: 1/2 Grain (Starch); 1 Lean Protein; 1/2 Vegetable.

ANUTRA® YOGURT SMOOTHIE

Makes 6 Servings

2 cups pineapple juice — unsweetened
1 cup strawberries — sliced
1 banana — sliced or
1 mango — diced or
1 papaya — diced
3 cups Anutra® Blueberry Yogurt
1/3 cup ANUTRA®
1 cup ice

Prepare fruit of choice. Combine all ingredients in a blender. Puree until thick and very smooth. Serve in a glass garnished with a whole strawberry and a mint sprig (optional).

To increase the nutrition, replace the pineapple juice with Anutra® Milk.

Nutrition per serving: 209 Calories; 3.8g Fat (16% calories from fat); 5.1g Protein; 39.2g Carbohydrate; 0mg Cholesterol; 72mg Sodium. Exchanges: 1-1/2 Grain (Starch); 1/2 Lean Protein; 1 Fruit.

ANUTRASIZED™ CHEDDAR OMELET WITH SPINACH AND ANUTRA® SOUR CREAM

Makes 1 Serving

OMELET:
1/2 cup 99% fat-free egg substitute or egg whites
1 tablespoon ANUTRA®
1 tablespoon Anutra® Cream Cheese
1 tablespoon Anutra® Milk
2 tablespoon water
2 tablespoons Anutra® Cheddar Shreds
vegetable cooking spray

FILLING:
1/2 cup thawed frozen spinach — drained
1 tablespoon Anutra® Sour Cream
1/4 teaspoon ground nutmeg

Mix and beat together all omelet ingredients until fluffy. Apply vegetable cooking spray to skillet heated to medium and add the egg mixture. Using a small spatula, run around the edges of the skillet, tipping the skillet so the uncooked egg from the center of the pan can run under the bottom of the cooked egg. Continue to do this until the egg in the center is a little moist, sprinkle the spinach in, top it with sour cream, sprinkle with nutmeg, then roll the omelet with three folds as you turn it onto the plate.

Nutrition per serving: 192 Calories; 7.3g Fat (34% calories from fat); 20.8g Protein; 13.5g Carbohydrate; 0mg Cholesterol; 601mg Sodium. Exchanges: 2-1/2 Lean Protein; 1 Vegetable; 1/2 Fat.

WHOLE GRAIN AND OAT ANUTRA® MILK PANCAKES

Makes 4 Servings

1 cup all-purpose flour
1/2 cup whole wheat flour
1/2 cup Quaker® oatmeal
1/4 cup ANUTRA®
1/2 cup sugar
1 teaspoon baking soda
2 teaspoons baking powder
3/4 cup Anutra® Milk
1/2 cup water
1/2 cup 99% fat-free egg substitute or egg whites
1/4 cup Anutra® Butter
1 teaspoon vanilla
Aunt Jemima® Lite syrup (optional)

Combine flour, ANUTRA®, oatmeal, salt, sugar, baking soda, and baking powder into a large mixing bowl. In a separate bowl, whisk together the Anutra® Milk, water, eggs, and Anutra® Butter. Add the wet ingredients to the dry. Stir with a spoon to combine. Lightly spray a griddle or skillet with cooking spray; heat until it is moderately hot. Drop the batter onto griddle, using a 1/3 measuring cup, leaving about 1 inch of space between pancakes. Cook the pancakes until the undersides are brown, the edges begin to dry, and bubbles begin to break the surface of the batter, about 1 - 2 minutes. Turn the pancakes and cook them until the second side is brown. Repeat using the remaining batter. Serve.

Top with Anutra® Butter, Aunt Jemima® Lite syrup, fresh fruit, or preserves.

Nutrition per serving: 405 Calories; 6.7g Fat (15% calories from fat); 13g Protein; 74.3g Carbohydrate; 0mg Cholesterol; 787mg Sodium. Exchanges: 3 Grain (Starch); 1/2 Lean Protein; 1-1/2 Fruit; 1/2 Fat; 1-1/2 Other Carbohydrates.

MY FAVORITE BREAKFAST - ANUTRASIZED™:

Makes _____ **Servings**

Ingredients:

_____   _____
_____   _____
_____   _____
_____   _____
_____   _____
_____   _____
_____   _____

Instructions:

_____
_____
_____
_____
_____
_____
_____
_____
_____
_____
_____
_____
_____
_____
_____

Nutrition per serving:
_____Calories;   _____g Fat (_____% Fat Cal);   _____g Protein;
_____g Carbohydrate;   _____mg Cholesterol;   _____mg Sodium.
Exchanges:
_____Grain (Starch);   _____Lean Protein;   _____Vegetable;
_____Fruit;   _____Other Carbohydrate

AnutraSize™

APPETIZERS

BLACK BEAN PANCAKES WITH HUMMUS MOUSSE & ANUTRA® BLUE CRUMBLES

Makes 8 Servings

MOUSSE:
1 tablespoon hummus (store bought or make your own)
2 tablespoons Anutra® Cream Cheese

TOPPING:
2 tablespoons Anutra® Blue Cheese Crumbles

PANCAKES:
1 can black beans, cooked - 15 ounce can/drained
1/2 cup ANUTRA®
1 cup water
1/2 cup Anutra® Milk
1-1/2 teaspoons honey
1 teaspoon jalapeño - minced
1 teaspoon cilantro - chopped
1/2 cup all-purpose flour
3/4 teaspoon baking powder
3/8 teaspoon baking soda
1/4 cup egg whites

For mousse: Puree ingredients in a food processor. Spoon into a crock, cover with plastic wrap, and refrigerate until serving time. For pancakes: drain and rinse all the black beans. Place 1/2 beans, honey, Anutra®, water and Anutra® Milk in processor. Puree. Transfer to a large bowl. Add the pepper and cilantro. Place in bowl with pureed mixture. In a medium sized bowl, combine the flour, baking powder, and baking soda. In another bowl, beat egg whites until stiff but not dry. Fold 1/3 of beaten egg whites into bean mixture. Slowly fold in remaining egg whites in 3 parts. Add the flour mixture to the bean mixture. Do not over-mix and deflate egg whites. Lightly spray a griddle or skillet with cooking spray; heat until moderately hot. Drop the batter onto griddle, using a 2 ounce ladle, leaving about 1 inch of space between pancakes. Cook the pancakes until the undersides are brown, the edges begin to dry, and bubbles begin to break the surface of the batter, about 1 - 2 minutes. Turn the pancakes and cook them until the second side is brown. Repeat using the remaining batter. Pipe mousse onto pancakes using pastry bag. Top with Anutra® Blue Cheese Crumbles. Serve immediately.

Nutrition per serving: 116 Calories; 3.3g Fat (26% calories from fat); 6.6g Protein; 16.1g Carbohydrate; 0mg Cholesterol; 195mg Sodium. Exchanges: 1 Grain (Starch); 1/2 Lean Protein.

PORT AND ANUTRA® CHEDDAR BALLS

Makes 8 Servings

1 cup Anutra® Cheddar Shreds
1/2 cup ANUTRA®
2 tablespoons port wine
2 teaspoons fresh parsley - chopped fine
3/4 cup water
1/4 cup chopped walnuts

Place Anutra® Shreds, Anutra®, water and port wine into a food processor or large bowl; blend together until smooth. Roll into desired size balls and roll into chopped walnuts. Cover with plastic wrap and refrigerate for 1 hour before serving.

This wine-rich spread can be served in a variety of ways: Spread it on celery or cucumber boats; roll it into a large ball; cover with crusted pecans and chill in wax paper until ready to serve; packed into raw mushroom caps; or layered on rye crackers. The spread will keep for up to two weeks if refrigerated, and the wine flavor will deepen.

Nutrition per serving: 87 Calories; 5.7g Fat (59% calories from fat); 5g Protein; 3.9g Carbohydrate; 0mg Cholesterol; 195mg Sodium. Exchanges: 1/2 Lean Protein; 1/2 Fat.

SPINACH AND ARTICHOKE
ANUTRA® CREAM CHEESE DIP

Makes 10 Servings

1/3 cup Anutra® Cream Cheese
8 ounces artichoke hearts - drained wt.
1/3 cup frozen chopped spinach - drained
2/3 cup ANUTRA®
1/2 teaspoon Tabasco® sauce
1/4 cup Anutra® Sour Cream
1 tablespoon garlic - chopped
1/4 teaspoon pepper
1/4 teaspoon salt
1/2 teaspoon lemon juice
1 cup water

Place all ingredients in food processor and blend until smooth.
Place in container and chill for 2 hours. Serve with crackers or
toasted breads.

Nutrition per serving: 64 Calories; 3.5g Fat (49% calories from fat); 3.7g Protein;
3.9g Carbohydrate; 0mg Cholesterol; 151mg Sodium. Exchanges: 1/2 Vegetable.

SUN-DRIED TOMATO AND ANUTRA®
MOZZARELLA APPETIZERS

Makes 10 Servings

1 pint cherry tomatoes
1/4 pound Anutra® Mozzarella "Chefs Award" - diced
1/2 cup ANUTRA®
1/2 cup water
1 tablespoon reduced fat balsamic dressing
1 garlic clove - minced
2 tablespoons fresh basil leaf - minced
1/4 cup sun-dried tomatoes
pinch black pepper

Soak sun-dried tomatoes in water for a few minutes according to directions on package. Dry, then mince. Cut mozzarella into 1/4-inch cubes. Chop fresh basil leaves finely. Mince garlic clove; use more garlic if preferred. Combine the cheese, Anutra®, water, basil, garlic, sun-dried tomatoes and black pepper in small bowl. Add the olive oil and blend well. Cover and refrigerate 1 hour to blend flavors. Just before serving, prepare cherry tomatoes by removing the stem end, cutting a thin slice from bottom of tomato to keep it setting straight and removing center from tomatoes with melon baller or small spoon. Sprinkle inside of tomatoes very lightly with salt and invert on paper towels to drain briefly. Stuff the tomatoes with the cheese mixture, garnish with small basil leaves and serve immediately.

Nutrition per serving: 76 Calories; 3.3g Fat (39% calories from fat); 4.5g Protein; 7.6g Carbohydrate; 0mg Cholesterol; 177mg Sodium. Exchanges: 1/2 Lean Protein; 1/2 Vegetable.

ANUTRA® FETA BRUSCHETTA
WITH SUN-DRIED TOMATOES

Makes 8 Servings

2 sun-dried tomatoes
2 tomatoes — peeled, seeded, chopped
2 tablespoons red onion — minced
2 garlic cloves — minced fine
1/4 cup ANUTRA®
1/2 cup water
1-1/2 teaspoons balsamic vinegar
2 teaspoons fresh basil — chopped
2 teaspoons fresh oregano — chopped
1/3 teaspoon ground black pepper
8 French bread slices — 1/2-inch thick
3 tablespoons Anutra® Feta Cheese Crumbles

Preheat oven to 350 degrees. Reconstitute the sun-dried tomatoes by placing them in a small bowl and pouring about one cup of boiling water over them. Let the tomatoes rest for 5 minutes. Drain the tomatoes and chop them finely. In a separate bowl, combine all ingredients, except the bread slices and the cheese, and set aside. Toast the bread slices in the oven until golden brown. Cool slightly. Top with tomato mixture, then with 1/2 teaspoon of Anutra® Feta Cheese Crumbles. Place back in oven for 2 - 3 minutes or until cheese has slightly melted.

Nutrition per serving: 128.6 Calories; 3.4g Fat (24% calories from fat); 5.2g Protein; 19.9g Carbohydrate; 0mg Cholesterol; 240mg Sodium. Exchanges: 1 Grain (Starch); 1/2 Vegetable.

ANUTRA® BLUE CHEESE CRUMBLE CROSTINI

Makes 12 Servings

1/2 cup Anutra® Blue Cheese Crumbles
1/3 cup ANUTRA®
2/3 cup water
1/4 cup Anutra® Cream Cheese — softened
1/2 tablespoon brandy
1/4 cup pecans — coarsely chopped
12 baguette slices

Preheat oven to 425 degrees. Thoroughly mix Anutra® cheeses (a food processor works best), Anutra® and water. Stir in brandy and pecans. Arrange bread slices on a baking sheet. Spread cheese mixture over bread slices. Bake until cheese is lightly browned (about 10 minutes). Serve immediately.

Nutrition per serving: 140 Calories; 5.8g Fat (37% calories from fat); 6.2g Protein; 16.4g Carbohydrate; 0mg Cholesterol; 319mg Sodium. Exchanges: 1 Grain (Starch); 1/2 Lean Protein; 1/2 Fat.

ANUTRA® CHEDDAR BAGUETTE MELTS

Makes 36 Servings

2 cups Anutra® Cheddar Shreds
4-1/2 ounces ripe olives — chopped
2 ounces pimientos — diced
4 green onions — finely chopped
2/3 cup ANUTRA®
1 cup water
1/2 cup Anutra® Cream Cheese
1-1/2 tablespoons prepared horseradish
1 large baguette — sliced diagonally

Mix together Anutra®, water, Anutra® Cheddar Shreds, olives, pimientos, green onions, Anutra® Cream Cheese, and horseradish. Spoon about 1 tablespoon cheese mixture onto each baguette slice. Broil until cheese starts to melt.

This topping can be made up to 2 days ahead, refrigerated, and used as needed.

Nutrition per serving: 91 Calories; 3.8g Fat (38% calories from fat); 4.4g Protein; 10.8g Carbohydrate; 0mg Cholesterol; 220mg Sodium. Exchanges: 1/2 Grain (Starch);1/2 Lean Protein.

ANUTRA® CHEDDAR JALAPEÑO QUESADILLAS

Makes 8 Servings

4 flour tortillas - 10-inch
1/4 cup fat-free refried beans
1/2 cup ANUTRA®
1 cup water
1 dash cumin
2 teaspoons fresh cilantro — diced
1/4 cup salsa
8 Anutra® Cheddar Jalapeño Slices

Heat non-stick skillet. Mix refried beans, Anutra®, water, cumin and fresh cilantro. Spread refried bean mixture over half of each flour tortilla. Place the Anutra® Slices over the beans, then place the salsa on the cheese. Fold bottom half on top. Heat in non-stick skillet on both sides until golden brown and cheese is melted. Cut each tortilla into 4 wedges and serve each person 2 wedges.

Nutrition per serving: 184 Calories; 6.8g Fat (33% calories from fat); 9.9g Protein; 20.9g Carbohydrate; 0mg Cholesterol; 693mg Sodium. Exchanges: 1/2 Grain (Starch); 1/2 Lean Protein; 1/2 Fat.

ANUTRA® CHEESY QUESADILLAS

Makes 12 Servings

1-1/2 cups Anutra® Shreds - Monterey Jack and Cheddar Blend
1/2 cup Anutra® Asiago Cheese Crumbles
6 medium 10-inch flour tortillas
3/4 cup ANUTRA®
6 green onions — diced
24 sprigs cilantro (optional)
vegetable cooking spray

In a small bowl, combine Anutra® cheese. Sprinkle one-sixth of the cheese mixture on 1 flour tortilla. Dot with diced green onions and 2 sprigs cilantro (if used)and Anutra® (1-2 tablespoons per tortilla). Cover with a second tortilla. Repeat with remaining tortillas. In a 12-inch non-stick skillet over medium-high heat, apply light layer of vegetable cooking spray. Cook stuffed tortillas, one at a time, until very lightly browned and crispy (about 3 minutes). Turn and cook second side until tortilla is lightly browned and cheese is melted (about 2 minutes). Remove from pan and reserve in a warm oven until all quesadillas are done. Cut each in 6 pieces at serving time and serve with salsa. Serves 12 as an hors d'oeuvre, 6 as a sandwich, or 6 as an accompaniment.

Quesadillas make excellent hors d'oeuvres or accompaniments to soup or salad. Serve with your favorite salsa.

Nutrition per serving: 191 Calories; 6.1g Fat (29% calories from fat); 9.7g Protein; 26.3g Carbohydrate; 0mg Cholesterol; 526mg Sodium. Exchanges: 1 Grain (Starch); 1/2 Lean Protein; 1 Vegetable; 1/2 Fat.

ANUTRA® CHILI DIP

Makes 10 Servings

1 small onion — diced
1 medium green pepper — diced
1 tablespoon olive oil
1 tablespoon garlic — chopped fine
1 tablespoon chili powder
2/3 cup ANUTRA®
1-1/3 cup water
1/2 teaspoon cayenne pepper
15-1/2 ounces tomatoes, canned — diced
15-1/2 ounces kidney beans, canned — small
1/2 cup ANUTRA® RAREBIT SAUCE (see recipe page 306)
1/2 cup Anutra® Cream Cheese
1/2 cup Anutra® Cheddar Shreds

Heat oil in medium sized sauce pan; add onions, peppers and garlic. Sauté for 2 minutes. Add diced tomatoes, kidney beans, chili powder, Anutra®, water and cayenne pepper. Cook for 12 minutes. Add rarebit sauce, Anutra® Cream Cheese, and Anutra® Shreds.

Nutrition per serving: 130 Calories; 4.9g Fat (34% calories from fat); 8.6g Protein; 15g Carbohydrate; 0mg Cholesterol; 473mg Sodium. Exchanges: 1/2 Grain (Starch); 1/2 Lean Protein; 1/2 Vegetable.

ANUTRA® HERBED CHEESE SPREAD ON RYE

Makes 16 Servings

8 ounces Anutra® Feta Cheese Crumbles
3/4 cup ANUTRA®
1 cup water
8 ounces Anutra® Cream Cheese
2 tablespoons Anutra® Sour Cream
1 garlic clove
1 tablespoon fresh chives — cut in 3-inch pieces
1/2 teaspoon fresh basil leaves — chopped
1 tablespoon fresh parsley — chopped
1/4 teaspoon fresh thyme — chopped
32 melba toast, rye

Add Anutra® Feta Cheese Crumbles Anutra® and water into food processor. Mash garlic clove with flat edge of knife or in garlic press and add to processor bowl. Add herbs; process just until herbs are chopped. Add Anutra® Cream Cheese and Sour Cream. Process until desired consistency, adding more sour cream for a softer spread. Serve with melba toast.

This recipe is excellent for stuffing raw vegetables such as celery, cherry tomatoes and pepper wedges. It also serves well with toasted focaccia bread.

Nutrition per serving: 124 Calories; 5.6g Fat (41% calories from fat); 7.8g Protein; 12g Carbohydrate; 0mg Cholesterol; 401mg Sodium. Exchanges: 1/2 Grain (Starch); 1 Lean Protein; 1/2 Fat.

ANUTRA® PARMESAN STUFFED MUSHROOMS

Makes 6 Servings

1/2 pound mushrooms
6 tablespoons Anutra® Parmesan Cheese
1/3 cup ANUTRA®
2/3 cup water
4 tablespoons Italian bread crumbs
1 tablespoon fresh parsley — chopped
garlic salt — to taste
black pepper — to taste

Remove stems from mushrooms and reserve. Wash mushrooms and leave moist. Combine half the cheese with the crumbs. Add Anutra®, water, garlic, salt and black pepper to your preference. Roll the moist mushrooms in the cheese mixture; place cup side up on shallow non-stick baking pan sprayed with cooking spray. Dry the stems and chop; add parsley and the remaining cheese. Spoon this mixture into the caps. Bake in preheated 475 degree oven 8-10 minutes or until browned.

Nutrition per serving: 77 Calories; 3.1g Fat (36% calories from fat); 5.5g Protein; 8g Carbohydrate; 0mg Cholesterol; 254mg Sodium. Exchanges: 1/2 Lean Protein; 1/2 Vegetable.

ANUTRA® ROASTED RED PEPPER DIP

Makes 8 Servings

1 medium red pepper — seeded
1 medium green pepper — seeded
1 small garlic clove
1/2 cup ANUTRA®
1 cup water
3 tablespoons Anutra® Cream Cheese
1/2 teaspoon balsamic vinegar
1 dash salt
2 pinches crushed red pepper

Cut peppers in half lengthwise; discard the seeds and membranes. Place the peppers, skin side up on a foil-lined baking sheet; flatten with palm of hand. Add garlic cloves to baking sheet. Broil 3 inches from heat for 4 minutes. Turn garlic over; broil 4 minutes or until garlic is blackened and charred. Remove garlic from baking pan; set aside. Broil peppers an additional 2 minutes or until blackened and charred. Place peppers in a zip-top heavy-duty plastic bag, and seal. Let stand for 15 minutes. Peel peppers and garlic; discard skins. Place the bell peppers Anutra®, water, and garlic in food processors; process until smooth scraping down sides of bowl once. Add Anutra® Cream Cheese and process until smooth. Spoon mixture into a bowl; stir in vinegar, salt, and pepper. Cover and chill. Serve with an assortment of vegetables or baked chips.

Nutrition per serving: 40 Calories; 2.6g Fat (59% calories from fat); 1.1g Protein; 3.3g Carbohydrate; 0mg Cholesterol; 75mg Sodium. Exchanges: Free

ANUTRA® SPINACH AND ARTICHOKE DIP

Makes 22 Servings

1/2 cup Anutra® Cream Cheese
8 ounces artichoke hearts — drained wt.
1 cup ANUTRA®
2 cups water
1 tablespoon low fat mayonnaise
4 ounces frozen chopped spinach — drained
3/4 teaspoon Tabasco® sauce
1/4 cup Anutra® Sour Cream
1-1/3 tablespoons chopped garlic
1/4 teaspoon pepper
1/2 teaspoon salt
3/4 teaspoon lemon juice

Place all ingredients in food processor and blend until smooth.
Place in container and chill for 2 hours. Serve with baked corn
chips.

Nutrition per serving: 47 Calories; 2.9g Fat (56% calories from fat); 2.5g Protein;
4.2g Carbohydrate; 0mg Cholesterol; 107mg Sodium. Exchanges: 1/2 Vegetable.

ANUTRA® VEGETABLE GUACAMOLE

Makes 8 Servings

1/2 cup fresh corn kernels
3 tablespoons red bell pepper — diced
3 tablespoons onion — diced
1 teaspoon jalapeño chile pepper — diced
1/2 teaspoon vegetable oil
1 teaspoon ground cumin
1-1/2 garlic cloves
2 avocados — pitted and chopped
1/2 cup ANUTRA®
3/4 cup water
2 teaspoons lemon juice
1/2 tomato — diced
2 teaspoons Anutra® Sour Cream
2 teaspoons cilantro — chopped

Preheat oven to 375 degrees. Place corn, peppers, onions, cumin, garlic, and oil in bowl and mix. Spread mixture on sheet pan and roast in oven for 8-10 minutes until corn is golden brown. Set aside to cool. Combine avocado, Anutra®, water tomato, Anutra® Sour Cream, and cilantro in bowl. Add vegetable mixture. Salt and pepper to taste. Chill for an hour. Serve.

Nutrition per serving: 107 Calories; 8.6g Fat (72% calories from fat); 2.3g Protein; 7.9g Carbohydrate; 0mg Cholesterol; 7mg Sodium. Exchanges: 1/2 Vegetable; 1-1/2 Fat.

ANUTRA® VEGETABLE PIZZA
7 INCH FOR APPETIZERS

Makes 8 Servings

2 pizza crusts (prebaked) -7 ounce
1/2 teaspoon olive oil
1/4 teaspoon chopped garlic
2 tablespoons zucchini — 1/4-inch diced
2 tablespoons yellow squash — 1/4-inch diced
2 tablespoons sliced mushrooms
2 tablespoons red bell peppers — 1/4-inch diced
2 tablespoons red onions — 1/4-inch diced
1 tablespoon balsamic vinegar
1 teaspoon basil
1 teaspoon oregano
1/2 cup pizza sauce — your favorite
1/2 cup ANUTRA®
1/2 cup water
2 teaspoons Anutra® Parmesan Cheese
1 cup Anutra® Mozzarella Shreds

Preheat oven to 450 degrees. Place a large sauté pan over a high heat. Add olive oil, and wait 30 seconds as pan heats. Add garlic, zucchini, yellow squash, mushrooms, onions and peppers stirring as needed. Cook for 3 minutes. Add balsamic vinegar, basil and oregano. Cook until vegetables are tender, about 3 more minutes. Remove from heat and set aside until needed. Add Anutra® and water to pizza sauce and spread pizza sauce on crust to the edges. Place half of the Anutra® Mozzarella Shreds over the sauce. Spread cooked vegetables over the shreds. Sprinkle Anutra® Parmesan topping over the vegetables. Place the rest of the moz-zarella on top of the vegetables and bake for 10-12 minutes or until the Anutra® Mozzarella is melted. Cut each pizza into 4 slices.

Nutrition per serving: 146 Calories; 5.4g Fat (33% calories from fat); 4.7g Protein; 12.6g Carbohydrate; 0mg Cholesterol; 122mg Sodium. Exchanges: 1/2 Grain (Starch); 1/2 Lean Protein; 1/2 Vegetable; 1/2 Fat.

MY FAVORITE APPETIZER - ANUTRASIZED™:

Makes _____ Servings

Ingredients:

_____   _____
_____   _____
_____   _____
_____   _____
_____   _____
_____   _____
_____   _____

Instructions:

_____
_____
_____
_____
_____
_____
_____
_____
_____
_____
_____
_____
_____
_____
_____

Nutrition per serving:
_____Calories;   _____g Fat (_____% Fat Cal);   _____g Protein;
_____g Carbohydrate;   _____mg Cholesterol;   _____mg Sodium.
Exchanges:
_____Grain (Starch);   _____Lean Protein;   _____Vegetable;
_____Fruit;   _____Other Carbohydrate

AnutraSize™

SALADS

ANUTRASIZED™ CAESAR SALAD

Makes 8 Servings

SALAD:
1 cup Anutra® Caesar Dressing
1 cup Anutra® Croutons
1/2 cup Anutra® Shreds -
  Parmesan, Mozzarella &
  Romano Blend
16 cups romaine lettuce — cut in 1
  inch pieces
1/2 cup ANUTRA®

ANUTRA® CROUTONS:
2 cups loaf Italian bread — cut
  into 1/2-inch cubes
1 tablespoon Anutra® Butter
1-1/2 tablespoons low sodium
  vegetable broth
2 teaspoons Anutra® Garlic Herb
  Parmesan
1/4 teaspoon garlic powder

"ANUTRASIZED™" CAESAR DRESSING:
1/2 cup Anutra® Sour Cream
1/4 cup Anutra® Cream Cheese
2 tablespoons red wine vinegar
1/2 cup Anutra® Parmesan Cheese
1 tablespoon Extra Virgin olive oil
1/2 teaspoon Worcestershire sauce
2 teaspoons dijon mustard
1 dash black pepper
2 anchovy fillets — optional
1/2 teaspoon garlic powder

DRESSING:
Place all ingredients in blender and mix until smooth. Chill for 30 minutes. Toss with greens as desired.

CROUTONS:
Heat oven to 350 degrees. Cut bread as described. Place in bowl. Heat butter and vegetable stock to liquid consistency. Pour on croutons, add Anutra® Herb Parmesan and garlic powder. Toss together using spatula. Place on non-stick baking pan. Place in oven for 5-7 minutes.

SALAD:
Place all ingredients in large mixing bowl. Combine all ingredients. Serve immediately.

Nutrition per serving: 303 Calories; 10.3g Fat (31% calories from fat); 15.2g Protein; 38.4g Carbohydrate; 0mg Cholesterol; 736mg Sodium. Exchanges: 2 Grain (Starch); 1 Lean Protein; 1/2 Vegetable; 1 Fat.

COUNTRY ANUTRA® POTATO SALAD

Makes 8 Servings

2 pounds red potatoes, whole — cooked & cooled
1/2 cup light ranch dressing
1/8 cup dijon mustard
1/4 cup Anutra® Sour Cream
1/2 cup onion — diced small
1/4 cup celery — diced small
2 tablespoons chopped parsley
2 tablespoons chopped chives
1/2 teaspoon white pepper
1 teaspoon salt
1 teaspoon Worcestershire sauce
6 egg whites — cooked and chopped
1/4 cup Anutra® Parmesan Cheese
1/2 cup Anutra®
1/4 cup water

Dice potatoes and place in large bowl. In a separate bowl, mix all other ingredients. Add mixture to potatoes and stir gently. Refrigerate for at least one hour and serve.

Nutrition per serving: 199 Calories; 6.9g Fat (31% calories from fat); 8.6g Protein; 26.8g Carbohydrate; 0mg Cholesterol; 584mg Sodium. Exchanges: 1-1/2 Grain (Starch); 1/2 Lean Protein.

CREAMY SOUR ANUTRASIZED™ BROCCOLI SALAD

Makes 6 Servings

2 pounds broccoli florets
1 tablespoon lemon juice
1/3 cup ANUTRA®
1/2 cup water
1/2 cup fat-free mayonnaise — or
  Nayonaise, tofu based vegetable dressing
1/2 cup Anutra® Sour Cream
1/2 teaspoon tarragon — crushed
4 scallions — minced
pinch black pepper

Steam or boil broccoli until bright green. Remove from cooking and rinse under cold water. Drain. Combine remaining ingredients in separate bowl. Toss in broccoli until well mixed. Cover and chill.

Nutrition per serving: 119 Calories; 4.6g Fat (35% calories from fat); 6.6g Protein; 17.4g Carbohydrate; 0mg Cholesterol; 315mg Sodium. Exchanges: 1/2 Lean Protein; 1-1/2 Vegetable; 1/2 Fat; 1/2 Other Carbohydrates.

LENTIL SALAD WITH ANUTRA®
FETA CRUMBLES

Makes 4 Servings

1-1/4 cups dried lentils
3 tablespoons fresh lemon juice
1 tablespoon olive oil
1/2 teaspoon dried thyme
1/4 cup ANUTRA®
1/2 cup water
1/4 teaspoon salt
1/8 teaspoon coarsely ground pepper
1 garlic clove — crushed
1-1/2 cups quartered cherry tomatoes
1 cup diced cucumber
1/2 cup Anutra® Feta Cheese Crumbles
1/3 cup thinly sliced celery

Place lentils in a large saucepan; cover with water 2 inches above
lentils and bring to a boil. Cover, reduce heat, and simmer 20 minutes or until tender. Drain well, and set aside. Combine lemon
juice and next 7 ingredients (lemon juice through garlic) in a medium bowl; stir with a wire whisk until blended. Add lentils, tomatoes, cucumber, Anutra® Feta Crumbles, and celery to lemon juice
mixture; toss gently to coat.

Nutrition per serving: 341 Calories; 9.2g Fat (24% calories from fat); 24.7g
Protein; 43.3g Carbohydrate; 0mg Cholesterol; 544mg Sodium. Exchanges: 2-1/2
Grain (Starch); 2-1/2 Lean Protein; 1 Vegetable; 1/2 Fat.

ROTINI WITH SPINACH, BEANS AND ANUTRA® ASIAGO SALAD

Makes 4 Servings

8 cups spinach leaves — coarsely chopped
6 ounces spiral shaped pasta — uncooked
1/4 cup ANUTRA®
1/2 cup water
2 tablespoons olive oil
1/4 teaspoon salt
1/4 teaspoon pepper
19 ounces canned cannellini beans — drained, or other white beans
2 garlic cloves — crushed
1/2 cup Anutra® Asiago Cheese Crumbles
fresh ground black pepper — optional

Cook pasta according to directions on box. Drain. Combine all ingredients in a large bowl and toss well. The warm pasta slightly wilts the spinach and softens the cheese during tossing.

You may substitute any of your favorite Anutra® Shreds in place of the Anutra® Asiago Crumbles.

Nutrition per serving: 489 Calories; 11.8g Fat (22% calories from fat); 25.8g Protein; 73g Carbohydrate; 0mg Cholesterol; 428mg Sodium. Exchanges: 4-1/2 Grain (Starch); 1 Lean Protein; 1 Vegetable; 1-1/2 Fat.

PEAR AND WATERCRESS SALAD
WITH ANUTRA® FETA

Makes 2 Servings

1-1/2 cups tightly packed torn red leaf lettuce
1/2 cup tightly packed trimmed watercress
1/2 cup red pear — thinly sliced
2 tablespoons Anutra® Feta Cheese Crumbles
1 tablespoon balsamic vinegar
2 tablespoons ANUTRA®
5 teaspoon water
1 teaspoon walnut oil or vegetable oil
1 teaspoon Dijon mustard
1 dash garlic powder
1 dash dried oregano

Divide leaf lettuce, watercress, and pear between 2 salad plates and sprinkle with Anutra® Feta Crumbles. Combine vinegar and next 6 ingredients in a bowl; stir well. Drizzle evenly over salads.

Nutrition per serving: 114 Calories; 6.2g Fat (49% calories from fat); 5.1g Protein; 11.6g Carbohydrate; 0mg Cholesterol; 234mg Sodium. Exchanges: 1/2 Lean Protein; 1/2 Vegetable; 1/2 Fruit; 1/2 Fat.

ANUTRA® MOZZARELLA ITALIAN PASTA SALAD

Makes 10 Servings

10 ounces pasta — Bowtie or Penne
2/3 cup ANUTRA®
1/4 red pepper — julienned
1/4 green pepper — julienned
1/4 yellow pepper — julienned
2 tablespoons sliced black olives — drained
1/4 cup red onion — julienned
1/2 cup sliced mushrooms
2 tablespoons chopped parsley
2 tablespoons sun-dried tomatoes — julienned
1/3 cup sliced green onions
1/3 cup Anutra® Parmesan Cheese
1 cup Anutra® Mozzarella Shreds
1 cup reduced fat Italian dressing
1-1/3 cup water

Cook pasta as directed on box. Chill. Place all ingredients in a large bowl and mix well. Serve and enjoy.

Nutrition per serving: 190 Calories; 4.7g Fat (22% calories from fat); 7 Protein; 30.9g Carbohydrate; 0mg Cholesterol; 475mg Sodium. Exchanges: 1-1/2 Grain (Starch); 1/2 Lean Meat; 1/2 Vegetable.

ANUTRA® PASTA SALAD

Makes 8 Servings

8 ounces pasta, uncooked — Bowtie or Penne
1/2 cup hearts of palm — cut diagonally
1 cup mushrooms — sliced
1/2 cup artichoke hearts — quartered
1/4 cup black olives — sliced
1 roasted red pepper — julienned
1/3 cup sun-dried tomatoes — julienned
1 medium carrot — shredded
1/2 cup ANUTRA®
1 cup water
1/2 cup reduced fat balsamic dressing
1/2 tablespoon oregano
1/2 teaspoon garlic powder
2 tablespoons Anutra® Parmesan Cheese
4 ounces Anutra® Mozzarella "Chefs Award" — cut into 1/2-inch cubes
2 Anutra® Provolone Slices — cut into 1/2-inch strips
1 tablespoon parsley — chopped fine
1 tablespoon chives — chopped
salt and pepper — to taste

Cook pasta as directed on box. Chill. In a bowl mix, place hearts of palm, mushrooms, artichoke hearts, black olives, roasted red peppers, sun-dried tomatoes, shredded carrots, Anutra®, water and balsamic vinaigrette dressing. Mix well and let marinate for 20 minutes. Add pasta, Anutra® Parmesan, mozzarella cubes, provolone strips, chives, parsley and garlic powder; mix well. Salt and pepper to taste. Refrigerate until ready to serve.

Nutrition per serving: 263 Calories; 6.3g Fat (22% calories from fat); 12g Protein; 40.6g Carbohydrate; 0mg Cholesterol; 617mg Sodium. Exchanges: 1-1/2 Grain (Starch); 1 Lean Protein; 1-1/2 Vegetable.

ANUTRA® PEPPER JACK AND CHEDDAR RANCH PASTA SALAD

Makes 10 Servings

8 ounces pasta, uncooked — Bowtie or Penne
2/3 cup ANUTRA®
1-1/3 cup water
1/2 cup sugar snap peas — julienned
1/2 cup sliced mushrooms
1/4 cup sliced green onions
1/2 cup sliced carrots
7 cherry tomatoes — quartered
1/4 cup diced celery
1/2 cup chopped broccoli
1/4 can sliced black olives
1 cup Anutra® Shreds - Pepper Jack and Cheddar Blend
1/2 teaspoon onion powder
1/4 teaspoon black pepper
1/2 teaspoon salt
3/4 cup light ranch dressing

Cook pasta as directed on box. Chill. In a large mixing bowl, place all ingredients and mix well. Chill for 20 minutes before serving.

Nutrition per serving: 221 Calories; 8.5g Fat (35% calories from fat); 8.6g Protein; 29g Carbohydrate; 0mg Cholesterol; 474mg Sodium. Exchanges: 1 Grain (Starch); 1/2 Lean Protein; 1 Vegetable.

ANUTRA® QUARTET BROCCOLI SLAW SALAD

Makes 6 Servings

1 pound broccoli cole slaw
1/4 cup dried cranberries — chopped
1/2 cup shredded carrots
1/2 cup chopped onion
1/4 cup Anutra® Blue Cheese Crumbles
1/3 cup green onion — sliced 1/8-inch thick
1/3 cup Anutra® Shreds - Parmesan, Mozzarella & Romano Blend
1/2 cup reduced fat balsamic dressing
1/3 cup ANUTRA®
2/3 cup water

Place all ingredients in a large bowl and mix well. Chill and serve.

Nutrition per serving: 77 Calories; 3.7g Fat (43% calories from fat); 5.2g Protein; 6.8g Carbohydrate; 0mg Cholesterol; 226mg Sodium. Exchanges: 1/2 Lean Protein; 1/2 Vegetable.

MY FAVORITE SALAD - ANUTRASIZED™:

Makes ____**Servings**

Ingredients:

_____   _____
_____   _____
_____   _____
_____   _____
_____   _____
_____   _____
_____   _____

Instructions:

_____
_____
_____
_____
_____
_____
_____
_____
_____
_____
_____
_____
_____
_____
_____
_____

Nutrition per serving:
____Calories;   ____g Fat (____% Fat Cal);   ____g Protein;
____g Carbohydrate; ____mg Cholesterol;   ____mg Sodium.
Exchanges:
____Grain (Starch);   ____Lean Protein;   ____Vegetable;
____Fruit;   ____Other Carbohydrate

AnutraSize™

SANDWICHES
& WRAPS

EGGPLANT AND ANUTRA® FETA PITAS

Makes 4 Servings

1 eggplant, cut 1/2-inch thick slices
vegetable cooking spray
4 pita bread pockets — 6-inch, cut in half
8 tomato slices — 1/2-inch-thick
1/4 cup Anutra® Feta Cheese Crumbles
1/4 cup chopped red onion
12 large fresh basil leaves — thinly sliced
1/4 cup ANUTRA®

Arrange eggplant in a single layer in a 13" x 9" baking dish coated with cooking spray. Cover; bake at 425 degrees for 10 minutes. Turn eggplant over; cook uncovered for 10 minutes. Let cool slightly.

Fill each pita half with 1 double sided Anutra® sprinkled eggplant slice, 1 tomato slice, 1/2 tablespoon of Anutra® Feta Crumbles, 1/2 tablespoon onion, and basil leaves. Serve.

Nutrition per serving: 280 Calories; 4.6g Fat (15% calories from fat); 11.1g Protein; 45.7g Carbohydrate; 0mg Cholesterol; 523mg Sodium. Exchanges: 2 Grain (Starch); 1/2 Lean Protein; 22 Vegetable.

GRILLED ANUTRA® CHEESE
SANDWICH

Makes 2 Servings

4 slices bread — focaccia, rye, whole wheat or multi-grain
4 Anutra® Cheddar Slices — or any Anutra® Slice flavor —
  or 1 cup of Anutra® Feta Crumbles
tomatoes (optional)
minced green bell peppers (optional)
vegetable cooking spray

Divide and place Anutra® Slices evenly on bread slices, sprinkle with green pepper and lay a slice of tomato on one of every two bread slices. Build sandwiches. Lightly coat non-stick cooking skillet with vegetable cooking spray and place on low heat. Add sandwiches. Brown and turn to brown other side (about 5 minutes per side). When cheese is melted, sandwich is done. If you have difficulty getting the cheese to melt all the way through, cover sandwich with a lid for a minute.

This is your basic grilled cheese sandwich Anutrasized™ which is a great fast food possibility! Try different breads such as focaccia, rye, french, or whole wheat. For a gourmet twist on this sandwich you can add sautéed mushrooms, onions, roasted eggplant, tomatoes or peppers.

Nutrition per serving: 214 Calories; 5.87.8g Fat (25% calories from fat); 12.2g Protein; 26.8g Carbohydrate; 0mg Cholesterol; 790mg Sodium. Exchanges: 1-1/2 Grain (Starch); 1 Lean Protein; 1-1/2 Fat.

ITALIAN BROCCOLI SLAW WRAP
ANUTRASIZED™

Makes 1 Serving

2 tablespoons low-fat Italian Dressing
1-1/2 cups broccoli cole slaw
3 tablespoons Anutra® Shreds - Parmesan, Mozzarella & Romano Blend
1 flour tortilla — 12-inch
1 tablespoon Anutra® Cream Cheese
1 tablespoon ANUTRA®
2 tablespoon water

In medium sized bowl, toss broccoli cole slaw, water Anutra® and low-fat Italian dressing. Fold in Anutra® Shreds. Lay tortilla flat and spread Anutra® Cream Cheese over top half of tortilla. Place broccoli slaw mixture across middle of tortilla. Fold sides approx 1 inch in and roll from the bottom up. Cut as desired.

Nutrition per serving: 273 Calories; 23.2g Fat (76% calories from fat); 13.4g Protein; 34.4g Carbohydrate; 0mg Cholesterol; 893mg Sodium. Exchanges: 1-1/2 Grain (Starch); 1/2 Lean Protein; 1/2 Fat.

OPEN-FACE PEPPER AND ANUTRA®
CHEESE MELTS

Makes 4 Servings

vegetable cooking spray
1 cup green bell pepper strips
1 tablespoon minced fresh basil
1 garlic clove — minced
1 medium onion, sliced and separated into rings
4 teaspoons stone-ground mustard
4 slices rye bread — toasted
4 tablespoons of ANUTRA®
8 slices unpeeled tomato — 1/4-inch thick, 2 medium
1 cup Anutra® Mozzarella Shreds

Coat a non-stick skillet with cooking spray; place over medium heat
until hot. Add next 4 ingredients; sauté 8 minutes or until tender.
Set aside and keep warm. Spread 1 teaspoon mustard over each
bread slice and sprinkle one tablespoon of Anutra®; place on a baking sheet. Top each with 2 slices tomato and 1/4 cup of Anutra®
Mozzarella Shreds. Broil 5 inches from heat until shreds melt. Top
each with about 1/3 cup bell pepper mixture.

You can also use any other flavor of Anutra® Shreds or Shred
Blends or any flavor of Anutra® Slices on your melt!

Nutrition per serving: 202 Calories; 6.5g Fat (29% calories from fat); 10.9g
Protein; 26.3g Carbohydrate; 0mg Cholesterol; 648mg Sodium. Exchanges: 1
Grain (Starch); 1 Lean Protein; 1 Vegetable.

ROASTED VEGETABLE PITAS WITH
ANUTRA® FETA DRESSING

Makes 4 Servings

1/4 cup Anutra® Feta Cheese Crumbles
1/4 cup Anutra® Sour Cream
1/4 cup Anutra® Milk
1/4 cup ANUTRA®
1/2 cup water
1 teaspoon prepared horseradish
1/4 teaspoon pepper
2 cups sliced zucchini
2 cups green bell pepper — cut into 1-inch pieces
1 teaspoon dried oregano
1 tablespoon olive oil
1/2 teaspoon salt
4 garlic cloves — minced
1 large tomato — cut into 8 wedges
1 large onion — cut into 8 wedges
vegetable cooking spray
2 pita bread pockets — 7-inch and halved

Combine first 7 ingredients in a small bowl; stir well and set aside.
In a medium bowl, combine zucchini and next 7 ingredients (zucchini through onion); toss gently. Spoon vegetable mixture onto a
broiler pan coated with cooking spray. Broil 10 minutes or until
tender and lightly browned, stirring occasionally. To serve, divide
vegetable mixture evenly between pita halves. Drizzle 2 tablespoons dressing over each sandwich.

You can also use eggplant, yellow squash, and red bell pepper in
this sandwich.

Nutrition per serving: 275 Calories; 9.4g Fat (31% calories from fat); 10.9g
Protein; 39.7g Carbohydrate; 0mg Cholesterol; 666mg Sodium. Exchanges: 1
Grain (Starch); 1 Lean Protein; 3 Vegetable; 1 Fat.

SOUTHWESTERN ANUTRA®
VEGETABLE WRAP

Makes 8 Servings

SALSA:
15 ounces black beans, cooked —
rinsed and drained
3 ears fresh corn — cut off the cob
1 onion — sliced 1/4-inch thick
24 ounces portabella mushrooms
— sliced 1/4-inch thick
1 teaspoon canola oil
1/4 cup fresh cilantro — chopped
fine
1 teaspoon southwestern seasoning
1/2 cup ANUTRA®

1 cup water
1 cup fat free ranch dressing
1 cup diced tomatoes
WRAP:
1 cup Anutra® Shred - Pepper Jack
and Cheddar Blend — 1/2 bag
8 flour tortillas — 12-inch
2 green peppers — sliced 1/4-inch
thick
4 tablespoons Anutra® Cream
Cheese
2 cups shredded lettuce

MUSHROOMS:
Rinse portabella mushrooms with water. Place in bowl and toss
with balsamic vinaigrette. Let set for 30 minutes. Place on roasting
pan and cook for 10-15 minutes until soft. Let cool.

SALSA:
Cut the corn off the cob, combine with sliced onion and portabella
mushrooms and toss with olive oil. Place on a non-stick baking pan
in oven for 20 minutes. In a bowl, place beans, cilantro, tomatoes,
roasted onion and corn. Set aside. In another bowl, mix ranch
dressing Anutra®, water, and southwestern seasoning. Mix well and
pour over salsa mix. Toss.

Place flour tortilla on a clean cutting board. Spread Anutra®
Cream Cheese across the top of the flour tortilla. Place approx 1/4
cup of salsa across the middle of the tortilla. Place 3 ounces
(approx 3-4 strips) of portabella mushroom strips on top of salsa.
Top with Anutra® Shreds - Pepper Jack and Cheddar Blend. Then
add 1 ounce of green pepper slices. Place 1/4 cup of shredded lettuce on top of green peppers. Folding in sides, roll like a burrito.
Cut in half. Serve.

Nutrition per serving: 313 Calories; 8.1g Fat (23% calories from fat); 17.7g
Protein; 49.2g Carbohydrate; 0mg Cholesterol; 467mg Sodium. Exchanges: 2-1/2
Grain (Starch); 1/2 Lean Protein; 1-1/2 Vegetable.

THE ANUTRA® BURGER!!

Makes 1 Serving

1 vegetable burger patty
1 hamburger bun, mixed grain
1 tablespoon ANUTRA®
1 Anutra® Cheddar Slice — or any Anutra® Slice
mustard — to taste (optional)
tomato ketchup — to taste (optional)
leaf lettuce (optional)
slice onion — (optional)
tomato slice — (optional)
1 tablespoon ANUTRA®
pickles — (optional)

Cook the vegetable burger patty according to directions on the box: oven, skillet or microwave. The Anutra® Slice goes on the burger about 15-20 seconds before removing from the heat. Sprinkle Anutra® over bottom bun, place the patty on it and garnish with whatever toppings satisfy your palate.

This is the Anutrasized™ American favorite.

Nutrition per serving: 310 Calories; 11.6g Fat (34% calories from fat); 24.1g Protein; 27.2g Carbohydrate; 0mg Cholesterol; 657mg Sodium. Exchanges: 1-1/2 Grain (Starch); 2-1/2 Lean Protein; 3 Fat.

THE ANUTRA® PATTY MELT

Makes 1 Serving

1 vegetable burger patty
1 pita bread pocket, 7-inch — or 2 slices bread of your choice
2 Anutra® Swiss Slices — or any Anutra® Slice
1 tablespoon ANUTRA®
2 tomato slices — 1/4-inch thick
condiments
vegetable cooking spray

Cook the Anutra® burger patty according to directions on the box: oven, skillet, microwave. Cut opening in pita large enough to insert filling. Set aside. Place one slice of tomato and Anutra® Cheese on each side of the patty and place inside pita bread round. Sprinkle Anutra® in pita Place in medium heated skillet coated with non-stick cooking spray. Let cook approx 1/2 to 1 minute on each side or until cheese melts. Garnish with condiments.

Nutrition per serving: 343 Calories; 11.8g Fat (31% calories from fat); 29.8g Protein; 30.8g Carbohydrate; 0mg Cholesterol; 923mg Sodium. Exchanges: 2 Grain (Starch); 3 Lean Protein; 1/2 Vegetable; 2 Fat.

VALERIE'S ANUTRA® CRUNCH GRILLED CHEESE

Makes 1 Serving

2 slices of your favorite bread
1 tablespoon Anutra® Butter
2 - 4 Anutra® Cheddar or American Slices - or any Anutra® Slice
sliced tomato (optional)

Coat one side of each slice of bread with Anutra® Butter; heat a non-stick pan over medium heat; add bread slices with Anutra® Butter side facing down; top each bread slice with one or two slices of Anutra® Slices. When Anutra® Slices are nearly melted, top each bread slice with a slice of tomato. Join both bread slices to make a sandwich and flip for a few seconds on each side and remove from pan.

Valerie's Anutra® Crunch Grilled Cheese is crunchy and delicious without any grease!

Nutrition per serving: 254 Calories; 8.8g Fat (32% calories from fat); 13.2g Protein; 28.8g Carbohydrate; 0mg Cholesterol; 910mg Sodium. Exchanges: 2 Grain (Starch); 1 Lean Protein; 2 Fat.

VEGETABLE ANUTRA® BURRITOS

Makes 6 Servings

16 ounces light red kidney beans — (1 can) drained
1/3 cup ANUTRA®
2/3 cup water
1 tablespoon chili powder
1/2 teaspoon garlic powder
1/2 cup frozen whole kernel corn — thawed
6 flour tortillas — (7-inch)
vegetable cooking spray
1 cup onion, thinly sliced
1/2 cup green bell pepper rings, thinly sliced
1/2 cup red bell pepper rings, thinly sliced
1-1/2 tablespoons lemon juice
1/3 cup mild salsa
14-1/2 ounces no-salt-added whole tomatoes —
*   (1 can) drained and chopped*
1 cup Anutra® Shreds - Pepper Jack and Cheddar Blend
1/2 cup Anutra® Sour Cream

Drain beans, reserving 1/4 cup liquid. In food processor bowl, add beans, reserved bean liquid, Anutra®, water, chili powder, and garlic powder. Process until smooth. Spoon bean mixture into a bowl; stir in corn. Set aside. Stack tortillas; wrap stack in damp paper towels and microwave at HIGH for 20 seconds. Spread 1/4 cup bean mixture down center of each tortilla, add 2 tablespoons of Anutra® Shreds on top of each mixture and roll up. Place tortillas seam side down in an 8-inch square baking dish coated with cooking spray. Cover and bake at 350 degrees for 30 minutes or until heated. Set aside; keep warm. Coat a large non-stick skillet with cooking spray; place over medium-high heat until hot. Add onion and next 3 ingredients; sauté 5 minutes or until crisp-tender. Reduce heat to medium. Add salsa and tomatoes; simmer 1 minute. Serve sauce over burritos. Garnish with Anutra® Sour Cream.

Nutrition per serving: 321 Calories; 9.3g Fat (26% calories from fat); 14.5g
Protein; 47.6g Carbohydrate; 0mg Cholesterol; 779mg Sodium. Exchanges: 2-1/2
Grain (Starch); 1 Lean Protein; 1-1/2 Vegetable; 1/2 Fat.

ANUTRA® MOZZARELLA AND TOMATO PITAS

Makes 6 Servings

4 medium ripe unpeeled tomatoes, cut into 1/4-inch slices
3/4 cup Anutra® Mozzarella Shreds
1 teaspoon olive oil
1/4 cup chopped fresh basil
1/3 cup ANUTRA®
2/3 cup water
1/2 cup red wine vinegar
1/4 teaspoon pepper
1/4 teaspoon salt
2 garlic cloves — minced
6 pita bread pockets — 6-inch
6 leaf lettuce leaves

Prepare tomato as described. Combine Anutra® Shreds and next 7 ingredients in a small bowl; stir well. Cover and chill 1 hour. Split open top half of each pita bread pocket, and line with a lettuce leaf. Fill each with 4 slices of tomato and 1/6 of Anutra® Mozzarella mix.

Nutrition per serving: 256 Calories; 5.1g Fat (18% calories from fat); 10.4g Protein; 43.4g Carbohydrate; 0mg Cholesterol; 604mg Sodium. Exchanges: 2 Grain (Starch); 1/2 Lean Protein; 1 Vegetable.

ANUTRA® PARMESAN, MOZZARELLA & ROMANO OPEN-FACED VEGETABLE MELT

Makes 4 Servings

1 teaspoon olive oil
1/2 cup thinly sliced onion
1 small zucchini — cut in 1/4-inch slices
2 garlic cloves — minced
1 cup chopped unpeeled tomato — fresh or canned
1/2 cup roasted red bell peppers — in jar, drained and coarsely chopped
1/2 teaspoon dried whole thyme
1/4 teaspoon pepper
3/4 cup Anutra® Shreds - Parmesan, Mozzarella & Romano Blend
1/4 cup ANUTRA®
1 loaf Italian bread — cut in half, split lengthwise and toasted
2 tablespoons Anutra® Parmesan Cheese

Heat oil in a medium size non-stick skillet over medium heat. Add onion, zucchini, and garlic; sauté 5 minutes or until tender. Add tomato and next 3 ingredients; cook 1 minute. Sprinkle 2 table-spoons of Anutra® Parmesan, Mozzarella, and Romano Shreds over each bread half; top each half with 1/2 cup vegetable mixture and 1 tablespoons of Anutra®. Sprinkle remaining 1/4 cup Anutra® Shreds and Anutra® Parmesan evenly over vegetable mixture. Broil 3 inches from heat 2 minutes or until shreds soften. Serve immediately.

This meatless sandwich resembles a French bread pizza.

Nutrition per serving: 192 Calories; 9.9g Fat (46% calories from fat); 10.5g Protein; 16.6g Carbohydrate; 15mg Cholesterol; 340mg Sodium. Exchanges: 1/2 Grain (Starch), 1 Lean Protein; 1 Vegetable; 1 Fat.

ANUTRA® PORTABELLA AND ROASTED PEPPER MOZZARELLA SANDWICH

Makes 4 Servings

vegetable cooking spray
6 cups portabella mushrooms — sliced 1/4-inch thick
1-1/2 teaspoons Worcestershire sauce
1 loaf Italian bread — split lengthwise, cut in 4 pieces (1-inch thick), lightly toasted
1/4 cup ANUTRA®
1/2 cup water-packed roasted red bell peppers, cut into thin peppers strips
4 Anutra® Mozzarella Slices
thyme sprigs (optional)

Coat a large non-stick skillet with cooking spray and place over medium-high heat until hot. Add mushrooms; sauté 4 minutes or until lightly browned. Remove from heat; stir in Worcestershire sauce. Spoon about 1/3 cup mushroom mixture and 1 tablespoon of Anutra® onto each bread slice; top each with one-fourth of the bell pepper strips and 1 Anutra® Mozzarella Slice. Place sandwiches on a baking sheet; and broil for 2 minutes or until cheese melts.

Nutrition per serving: 179 Calories; 5.1g Fat (26% calories from fat); 20.5g Protein; 31.8g Carbohydrate; 0mg Cholesterol; 454mg Sodium. Exchanges: 1 Grain (Starch), 1/2 Lean Protein; 2-1/2 Vegetable.

MY FAVORITE SANDWICH - ANUTRASIZED™:

Makes _____**Servings**

Ingredients:

_____   _____
_____   _____
_____   _____
_____   _____
_____   _____
_____   _____
_____   _____

Instructions:

_____
_____
_____
_____
_____
_____
_____
_____
_____
_____
_____
_____
_____
_____
_____

Nutrition per serving:
_____Calories;   _____g Fat (_____% Fat Cal);   _____g Protein;
_____g Carbohydrate;   _____mg Cholesterol;   _____mg Sodium.
Exchanges:
_____Grain (Starch);   _____Lean Protein;   _____Vegetable;
_____Fruit;   _____Other Carbohydrate

MY FAVORITE WRAP - ANUTRASIZED™:

Makes _____ **Servings**

Ingredients:

_____   _____
_____   _____
_____   _____
_____   _____
_____   _____
_____   _____
_____   _____

Instructions:

_____
_____
_____
_____
_____
_____
_____
_____
_____
_____
_____
_____
_____
_____

Nutrition per serving:
_____Calories;   _____g Fat (_____% Fat Cal);   _____g Protein;
_____g Carbohydrate; _____mg Cholesterol;   _____mg Sodium.
Exchanges:
_____Grain (Starch); _____Lean Protein;   _____Vegetable;
_____Fruit;   _____Other Carbohydrate

AnutraSize™

SOUPS, CHOWDERS
& CHILI

ANUTRASIZED™ IDAHO POTATO
AND CORN CHOWDER

Makes 8 Servings

4 cups Idaho potatoes — cut into 1/2-inch cubes
1/2 cup ANUTRA®
1 cup water
2 cups onion — chopped
3 cups low sodium vegetable broth
1 teaspoon dried parsley
2 teaspoons garlic powder
1/4 teaspoon pepper
1 cup creamed corn
1 cup low sodium canned corn — drained
1-1/2 cups Anutra® Milk

In a medium saucepan, combine the potatoes, onions, Anutra®,
water and one cup of vegetable broth. Bring to a boil for 5 minutes.
Remove pan from heat, place mixture into food processor and
puree. Return the pureed mixture to the saucepan, stir in the rest
of ingredients and heat thoroughly.

Nutrition per serving: 222 Calories; 3g Fat (12% calories from fat); 11.1g Protein;
41.4g Carbohydrate; 0mg Cholesterol; 227mg Sodium. Exchanges: 2-1/2 Grain
(Starch); 1/2 Lean Protein; 1/2 Vegetable.

CREAMY ANUTRA® CARROT SOUP

Makes 6 Servings

1 pound carrots — peeled and chopped
1 medium potato — peeled and chopped
1/3 cup ANUTRA®
2/3 cup water
1/2 cup Anutra® Butter
1/2 cup Anutra® Milk
1/4 teaspoon fresh ground pepper
3 cups low sodium vegetable broth
1/4 cup Anutra® Sour Cream — for garnish
sprigs of fresh parsley or cilantro — for garnish

In a medium saucepan over medium-low heat, add carrots, potatoes Anutra®, water and Anutra® Milk to pan; cover and simmer until vegetables are easily pierced with a sharp knife (about 25 minutes). Puree carrots and potato in a blender or food processor with Anutra® Butter and pepper. Return to saucepan and stir in broth. Place over medium heat and cook until warm. Serve immediately. Garnish each serving with a tablespoon of Anutra® Sour Cream and a sprig of fresh herb.

You can use this same recipe to make creamy cauliflower or broccoli soup. Just substitute the carrots with cauliflower or broccoli.

Nutrition per serving: 204 Calories; 7.4g Fat (33% calories from fat); 10.9g Protein; 25.3g Carbohydrate; 0mg Cholesterol; 350mg Sodium. Exchanges: 1 Grain (Starch); 1 Lean Protein; 1-1/2 Vegetable; 1 Fat.

EASY CHEESY ANUTRA® EGGPLANT SOUP

Makes 8 Servings

1/2 tablespoon olive oil
1 pound portabella mushrooms — cut in 1/2-inch cubes
1 large onion — chopped
1 large garlic clove — minced
1-1/2 pounds eggplant (1 medium), unpeeled — minced
2 medium carrots — shredded
1 green pepper — cut in 2-inch strips
28 ounces canned tomatoes — liquid reserved
1/2 cup ANUTRA®
1 cup water
1 teaspoon sugar
1 teaspoon dried basil
1/2 teaspoon ground nutmeg
1/4 teaspoon fresh ground pepper
1/2 cup Anutra® Butter
2-1/2 cups low sodium vegetable broth
1 cup Anutra® Mozzarella Shreds
1/2 cup chopped parsley
salt — to taste
3 tablespoons Anutra® Parmesan cheese — for garnish

In a large pot over medium heat, heat oil and cook portabella mushrooms and onion. Add garlic, eggplant, carrots, and green pepper. Cook, stirring occasionally, until eggplant browns lightly. Stir in tomatoes and their liquid, salt, sugar, basil, nutmeg, pepper, Anutra® Butter, Anutra®, water and vegetable broth. Bring to a boil over medium-high heat, reduce heat to low, cover, and simmer until the eggplant is very tender (45 to 50 minutes). Fold in 1 cup of Anutra® Mozzarella Shreds. Stir in parsley. Season with salt if desired. Top each with one teaspoon of Anutra® Parmesan.

Nutrition per serving: 196.8 Calories; 8.2g Fat (38% calories from fat); 14.7g Protein; 21.6g Carbohydrate; 0mg Cholesterol; 679mg Sodium. Exchanges: 1/2 Grain (Starch); 1/2 Lean Protein; 3 Vegetable; 1/2 Fat.

MINESTRONE SOUP WITH ANUTRA®
PARMESAN, MOZZARELLA & ROMANO

Makes 8 Servings

15 ounces low sodium kidney beans, canned — undrained
1/2 cup ANUTRA®
1 cup water
15 ounces navy beans, canned — drained
2-1/2 cups low sodium vegetable broth
1-1/2 cups zucchini — diced
1 cup leek — chopped
3/4 cup sliced celery
1/2 cup dry red wine
1 teaspoon Italian seasoning
1 garlic clove — minced
8 ounces no-salt-added tomato sauce
1/2 cup elbow macaroni — uncooked
1 cup tomatoes, low sodium — diced
1 cup Anutra® Shreds - Parmesan, Mozzarella & Romano Blend

Place half of kidney beans, Anutra® and water in a food processor
and process until smooth. Spoon bean puree into a medium sized
stock pot, stir in navy beans, stock, and the next 8 ingredients (stock
through tomato sauce). Bring to a boil; cover, reduce heat, and
simmer for 20 minutes. Stir in the elbow macaroni; cook, uncovered, an additional 10 minutes or until tender. Pour into bowls and
top each with 2 tablespoons of Anutra® Parmesan, Mozzarella, &
Romano Shreds.

Nutrition per serving: 230 Calories; 4.1g Fat (16% calories from fat); 16.1g
Protein; 32.6g Carbohydrate; 0mg Cholesterol; 554mg Sodium. Exchanges: 1-1/2
Grain (Starch); 1 Lean Protein; 1-1/2 Vegetable.

TORTILLA AND ANUTRA® CHEDDAR TOMATO SOUP

Makes 6 Servings

1/2 tablespoon olive oil
1 medium onion — diced small
1 small garlic clove — minced
1/2 teaspoon ground cumin
2 green chilies — finely chopped
1-1/2 cups tomato sauce
1/3 cup ANUTRA®
2 cups low sodium vegetable broth
1-2/3 cups water
4 ounces Anutra® Cheddar "Chefs Award" — cut in 1/2-inch cubes
1/2 cup Anutra® Sour Cream
4 ounces baked tortilla chips

In a medium saucepan, heat olive oil over medium heat. Add onion and sauté until soft, but not browned. Mix in garlic and cumin; add green chilies, tomato sauce, stock, Anutra® and water. Bring to a boil; cover, reduce heat, and simmer for 10 minutes. Place baked tortilla chips in soup bowls. Top with Anutra® Cheddar Chefs Award cubes. Ladle hot soup over baked tortilla chips and cheese and serve at once. Spoon a tablespoon of Anutra® Sour Cream in each bowl.

Anutra® Pepper Jack "Chefs Award" also works well with this recipe.

Nutrition per serving: 230 Calories; 8.1g Fat (32% calories from fat); 12.9g Protein; 29g Carbohydrate; 0mg Cholesterol; 670mg Sodium. Exchanges: 1 Grain (Starch); 1-1/2 Lean Protein; 1-1/2 Vegetable; 1/2 Fat.

ANUTRA® CREAM OF MUSHROOM SOUP

Makes 6 Servings

3 cups mushrooms — sliced
3 cups portabella mushrooms — chopped
1/2 medium onion — sliced
1 tablespoon olive oil
3 tablespoons water
1-1/2 teaspoons garlic clove — chopped fine
1/3 cup ANUTRA®
2/3 cup water
1-1/2 pints Anutra® Milk
1 cup low-sodium vegetable stock
1/4 teaspoon salt
1/4 teaspoon black pepper
1-1/2 tablespoons cornstarch
1-1/2 tablespoons water

Heat oil on high heat, sauté mushrooms and onions until mushrooms are soft. Add 3 tablespoons of water, continue to cook. Add garlic and lower heat to medium. Cook for one minute and add Anutra® Milk, Anutra®. and water. Cook for 10 minutes. Puree with hand blender until all large pieces are gone. Add vegetable stock, salt, pepper and cook 15 more minutes. Mix cornstarch and 2 tablespoons water. When soup is boiling, whisk in cornstarch quickly (so no lumps form). Cook for 10 more minutes. Serve.

Nutrition per serving: 138 Calories; 5.8g Fat (38% calories from fat); 11.2g Protein; 18g Carbohydrate; 0mg Cholesterol; 174mg Sodium. Exchanges: 1/2 Grain (Starch); 1/2 Lean Protein; 1-1/2 Vegetable; 1/2 Fat.

ANUTRA® CREAM OF TOMATO SOUP

Makes 4 Servings

2 teaspoons olive oil
1 medium onion — diced
1 pound canned tomatoes — 2 cans
1/2 teaspoon chopped garlic
1 teaspoon fresh basil — chopped
1 tablespoon tomato paste
3 cups Anutra® Milk
1/4 cup ANUTRA®
1/2 cup water

In a sauce pan, sauté onion in oil for 3 minutes or until transparent. Add tomatoes and garlic, continuing to sauté for 2-3 minutes. Add basil, salt, and pepper. Blend in Anutra® Milk, Anutra® and water. Cook stirring constantly for 1 minute. Remove from heat and cool briefly. Transfer to a food processor and puree until smooth. Serve hot or chilled.

Nutrition per serving: 170 Calories; 6.5g Fat (34% calories from fat); 9.4g Protein; 20.7g Carbohydrate; 0mg Cholesterol; 373mg Sodium. Exchanges: 1 Grain (Starch); 1 Lean Protein; 1-1/2 Vegetable; 1/2 Fat.

ANUTRA® MONTEREY JACK
THREE BEAN CHILI

Makes 8 Servings

1 cup chopped onion
1 clove garlic — minced fine
1/2 tablespoon olive oil
1/2 cup low sodium vegetable broth
1 cup black beans, cooked — 1/2-inch cubes
1 pint low sodium kidney beans, canned — rinsed and drained
1 cup great northern beans, canned
3 cups diced tomatoes, peeled, canned, use juice
2 tablespoons fresh cilantro — chopped
1 tablespoon dried basil
5-1/2 teaspoons chili powder
1 cup corn, canned — rinsed and drained
1/2 cup ANUTRA®
1 cup water
2 cups Anutra® Shreds - Monterey Jack and Cheddar Blend -
  (1- 8 ounce bag)

In a large pot, sauté onions and garlic in olive oil stirring until onions are translucent. Stir in remaining ingredients, except Anutra® Shreds. Heat to a boil. Reduce heat and simmer for 30 minutes. Stir occasionally. When finished cooking, stir in the bag of shreds or place 1/4 cup on each serving.

Nutrition per serving: 269 Calories; 6.8g Fat (23% calories from fat); 17.2g Protein; 38.2g Carbohydrate; 0mg Cholesterol; 591mg Sodium. Exchanges: 2 Grain (Starch); 1 Lean Protein; 1 Vegetable.

ANUTRA® PEPPER JACK AND CORN CHOWDER

Makes 6 Servings

vegetable cooking spray
1/3 cup ANUTRA®
2/3 cup water
1 cup chopped onion
1 cup vegetable broth — canned
1 cup chopped cauliflower
1/2 cup sliced carrot
1/2 cup sliced celery
1/2 cup sliced green beans
1 jalapeño pepper — halved lengthwise
1/4 cup all-purpose flour
3 cups Anutra® Milk
1/4 teaspoon white pepper
1 dash ground red pepper
11 ounces whole-kernel corn — drained
2/3 cup Anutra® Shreds - Pepper Jack and Cheddar Blend

Coat a large saucepan with cooking spray; place over medium heat until hot. Add onion; sauté 5 minutes or until tender. Add broth, Anutra®, water and the next 5 ingredients (broth through jalapeño pepper); bring to a boil. Cover, reduce heat, and simmer 20 minutes or until vegetables are tender. Place flour in a medium bowl. Gradually add Anutra® Milk, stirring with a wire whisk until blended. Add Anutra® Milk mixture, white pepper, red pepper, and corn to pan; stir well. Cook over medium heat 7 minutes or until thickened, stirring constantly. Discard jalapeño pepper.

To serve, ladle into individual bowls; sprinkle with Anutra® Pepper Jack and Cheddar Shreds.

Nutrition per serving: 227 Calories; 5.5g Fat (22% calories from fat); 12.4g Protein; 34.5g Carbohydrate; 0mg Cholesterol; 534mg Sodium. Exchanges: 2 Grain (Starch); 1 Lean Protein; 1 Vegetable.

ANUTRA® PEPPER JACK AND BROCCOLI SOUP

Makes 4 Servings

1 cup Anutra® Milk
1/4 cup ANUTRA®
1/2 cup water
16 ounces low sodium vegetable broth
4 Anutra® Pepper Jack Slices
4 Anutra® Cheddar Slices
2 tablespoons Anutra® Parmesan Cheese
1 cup broccoli florets

Place Anutra® Milk, Anutra®, water and vegetable stock in a sauce pan on medium heat. Once the mixture is warm, start adding the Anutra® Slices one at a time. Whisking until they are completely melted. Add Anutra® Parmesan topping and stir well. Add broccoli florets and cook for 3-5 minutes. Serve and enjoy.

Nutrition per serving: 174 Calories; 7.1g Fat (37% calories from fat); 18.3g Protein; 9.4g Carbohydrate; 0mg Cholesterol; 739mg Sodium. Exchanges: 1/2 Grain (Starch); 2 Lean Protein; 1 Fat.

ANUTRA® SOUTHWESTERN BLACK BEAN CHILI

Makes 8 Servings

1/4 cup dry cooking sherry
1 tablespoon olive oil
2 cups chopped onion
1/2 cup chopped celery
1/2 cup chopped carrot
1/2 cup seeded and chopped red bell pepper
4 cups cooked black beans — rinsed and drained, canned
1 cup low sodium vegetable broth
1/2 cup ANUTRA®
1 cup water
1 cup Anutra® Milk
2 tablespoons minced garlic
1 cup chopped tomatoes
2 teaspoons ground cumin
4 teaspoons chili powder — or to taste
1/2 teaspoon dried oregano
1/4 cup chopped cilantro
2 tablespoons honey
2 tablespoons tomato paste
2 cups Anutra® Shreds - Monterey Jack and Cheddar Blend
    (1 cup for garnish)
grated onion (for garnish)

In a large, heavy pot, heat cooking sherry and oil over medium heat and sauté onions until soft but not browned. Add celery, carrot, and bell pepper and sauté 5 minutes, stirring frequently. Add remaining ingredients, except garnishes, and bring to a boil. Lower heat and simmer for 45 minutes to 1 hour, covered. Chili should be thick. Fold in 1/2 of the Anutra® Shreds. Garnish with grated onion and other half of the Anutra® Shreds.

Nutrition per serving: 313 Calories; 8.5g Fat (24% calories from fat); 17.9g Protein; 42.1g Carbohydrate; 0mg Cholesterol; 673mg Sodium. Exchanges: 2 Grain (Starch); 1-1/2 Lean Protein; 1 Vegetable; 1/2 Fat; 1/2 Other Carbohydrates.

MY FAVORITE SOUP RECIPE- ANUTRASIZED™:

Makes _____ Servings

Ingredients:

_____   _____
_____   _____
_____   _____
_____   _____
_____   _____
_____   _____
_____   _____

Instructions:

_____
_____
_____
_____
_____
_____
_____
_____
_____
_____
_____
_____
_____
_____
_____
_____
_____

Nutrition per serving:
_____Calories;   _____g Fat (_____% Fat Cal);   _____g Protein;
_____g Carbohydrate;   _____mg Cholesterol;   _____mg Sodium.
Exchanges:
_____Grain (Starch);   _____Lean Protein;   _____Vegetable;
_____Fruit;   _____Other Carbohydrate

MY FAVORITE CHILI/CHOWDER - ANUTRASIZED™:

Makes _____ Servings

Ingredients:

_____   _____
_____   _____
_____   _____
_____   _____
_____   _____
_____   _____
_____   _____

Instructions:

_____
_____
_____
_____
_____
_____
_____
_____
_____
_____
_____
_____
_____
_____

Nutrition per serving:
_____Calories; _____g Fat (_____% Fat Cal); _____g Protein;
_____g Carbohydrate; _____mg Cholesterol; _____mg Sodium.
Exchanges:
_____Grain (Starch); _____Lean Protein; _____Vegetable;
_____Fruit; _____Other Carbohydrate

AnutraSize™

ENTRÉES

ANUTRASIZED™ PENNE PASTA A LA ANG'ELINO

Makes 8 Servings

6 tablespoons olive oil
6 garlic cloves
1 teaspoon crushed red pepper
24 ounces cannellini beans, canned in liquid
1/2 cup ANUTRA®
1 cup water
1 pound penne pasta
3 bunches broccoli florets
1 pound mushrooms — button
1 teaspoon garlic powder
1 tablespoon olive oil
2 tablespoons balsamic vinegar
1/2 cup Anutra® Shreds - Parmesan, Mozzarella & Romano Blend
pinch salt and pepper

Place mushrooms, garlic powder, balsamic vinegar, and olive in a small bowl. Toss and set aside to marinate. Heat large sauté pan to medium-high heat. Add olive oil, sauté garlic and crushed red pepper. Add cannellini beans, Anutra® and water bring to boil stirring constantly. Turn heat down to low and let simmer and thicken. Keep warm. In another medium stock pot, cook pasta according to directions adding broccoli 4 minutes before draining water. Add hot pasta mixture to sauce and toss. Sauté marinated mushrooms. Plate pasta and top with mushrooms and Anutra® Shreds.

Nutrition per serving: 384 Calories; 15.8g Fat (37% calories from fat); 12g Protein; 50.3g Carbohydrate; 0mg Cholesterol; 109mg Sodium. Exchanges: 3 Grain (Starch); 1/2 Lean Protein; 1 Vegetable; 2-1/2 Fat.

AUNT VIRGINIA'S ZUCCHINI CASSEROLE

Makes 6 Servings

2 pounds zucchini
1/3 cup ANUTRA®
1/3 cup water
1/2 teaspoon salt
1/4 teaspoon pepper
1/2 teaspoon garlic powder
1 teaspoon dried basil
1 cup all-purpose flour
1 cup Anutra® Shreds - Parmesan, Mozzarella & Romano Blend
1 tablespoon olive oil
2 tablespoons bread crumbs
2 tablespoons Anutra® Parmesan Cheese

Cut zucchini into 1 inch slices (if large remove center pulp).
Combine flour, salt, pepper, garlic powder, basil, and Anutra®
Shreds. Add to zucchini slices. Add olive oil. Place zucchini mixture in greased baking pan. Combine bread crumbs, Anutra®,
water and Anutra® Parmesan. Top casserole. Bake at 350 degrees
for 45 minutes.

Nutrition per serving: 202 Calories; 7.1g Fat (32% calories from fat); 10.3g
Protein; 25.9g Carbohydrate; 0mg Cholesterol; 493mg Sodium. Exchanges: 1
Grain (Starch); 1 Lean Protein; 1 Vegetable; 1/2 Fat.

AUNT VIRGINIA'S EGGPLANT
ANUTRA® PARMESAN

Makes 8 Servings

2 eggplants, whole — sliced 1/2-inch thick
1 cup all-purpose flour
1/2 teaspoon salt
1/4 teaspoon pepper
1/2 teaspoon garlic powder
1/2 cup ANUTRA®
1-1/2 tablespoons olive oil
1 teaspoon dried basil
8 ounces tomato sauce
2 cups Anutra® Shreds - Parmesan, Mozzarella & Romano Blend

Cut eggplant into 1/2" slices; salt slices and let sit for 1/2 hour.
Combine flour mixture and next 5 ingredients. Rinse and pat dry.
Dredge eggplant, in flour mixture. Shake off excess. Heat oil in a
medium skillet, then add eggplant; do not over-lap them. Brown
one side, turn and brown the other side. Layer in baking pan with
tomato sauce, basil, and Anutra® Shreds between layers and on top.
Do not exceed two layers. Cover with foil and bake at 350 degrees
for 45 minutes.

Nutrition per serving: 206 Calories; 7.9g Fat (35% calories from fat); 10.2g
Protein; 25.2g Carbohydrate; 0mg Cholesterol; 608mg Sodium. Exchanges: 1
Grain (Starch); 1 Lean Protein; 1-1/2 Vegetable; 1/2 Fat.

AUNT VIRGINIA'S POTATO
AU ANUTRA® GRATIN

Makes 4 Servings

2 tablespoons Anutra® Butter
2 tablespoons all-purpose flour
1/4 cup ANUTRA®
1/2 cup water
1 cup Anutra® Milk
pinch salt
1 cup Anutra® Cheddar Shreds
2 cups potatoes, diced
1/4 cup bread crumbs
1/4 teaspoon paprika
1/2 teaspoon onion powder
2 tablespoons Anutra® Butter

In medium sauce pan, melt 2 tablespoons of Anutra® Butter over low heat. Add flour blending over low heat. Add Anutra® Milk, Anutra®, water and salt cooking and stirring until thickened and smooth. Add Anutra® Cheddar Shreds or Anutra® Shred flavor of choice stirring until melted. Add diced potatoes until well combined. Place in lightly sprayed 2 quart baking dish. Combine bread crumbs, paprika, and onion powder. Top casserole. Add dots of Anutra® Butter to top of casserole and bake at 350 degrees until brown.

Nutrition per serving: 268 Calories; 9.1g Fat (31% calories from fat); 13.5g Protein; 32.5g Carbohydrate; 0mg Cholesterol; 624mg Sodium. Exchanges: 2 Grain (Starch); 1-1/2 Lean Protein; 1/2 Fat.

AUNT VIRGINIA'S ANUTRA®
MACARONI AND CHEESE

Makes 4 Servings

2 cups Anutra® Milk
1/4 cup ANUTRA®
1/2 cup water
1-1/2 tablespoons corn starch
2 cups Anutra® Cheddar Shreds
1-1/2 cups elbow macaroni
pinch salt and pepper
vegetable cooking spray

In medium sized sauce pan, combine Anutra® Milk, Anutra®, water, corn starch, salt and pepper. Heat until it starts to thicken. Add Anutra® Cheddar Shreds and cook until cheddar has melted. Cook macaroni according to directions on box. Drain macaroni and combine with sauce. Place in lightly vegetable sprayed baking dish at 350 degrees for 35 minutes.

Nutrition per serving: 281 Calories; 9.6g Fat (31% calories from fat); 20.2g Protein; 28.5g Carbohydrate; 0mg Cholesterol; 847mg Sodium. Exchanges: 1-1/2 Grain (Starch); 2-1/2 Lean Protein.

BAKED POTATOES STUFFED WITH ANUTRA® PARMESAN

Makes 6 Servings

6 large Idaho potatoes
6 tablespoons Anutra® Butter
1/3 cup ANUTRA®
1/2 cup water
1 package frozen spinach — thawed
1-1/4 cups Anutra® Parmesan Cheese
1-3/4 cups sliced mushrooms
salt and pepper

Bake potatoes, cut in half and scoop out pulp with a spoon. Place pulp in a bowl with two-thirds of the Anutra® Butter. Place potato shells in a baking dish, set aside. Spray heated skillet with vegetable cooking spray and cook mushrooms. Microwave frozen spinach until just thawed, then drain completely. Mash and blend potato and rest of Anutra® Butter together until well-blended; add Anutra® Parmesan, spinach Anutra®, water and mushrooms. Add extra seasoning if desired. Spoon mixture back into potato shells and place in 350 degree oven for another 15 minutes, until heated through. Serve immediately. For a main dish, two halves make a serving.

For a cheesier potato, try using any flavor of Anutra® Shreds to this recipe in place of the Anutra® Parmesan Cheese.

Nutrition per serving: 448 Calories; 8.2g Fat (16% calories from fat); 22.1g Protein; 74.8g Carbohydrate; 0mg Cholesterol; 598mg Sodium. Exchanges: 4-1/2 Grain (Starch); 1-1/2 Lean Protein; 1 Vegetable; 1/2 Fat.

BAKED VEGETABLES AU ANUTRA® GRATIN

Makes 8 Servings

1 tablespoon olive oil
1 onion — chopped
1 cup sliced mushrooms
1 large carrot, sliced the length of the carrot,
  each slice about 1/4-inch wide
1 zucchini sliced into long thin strips
2-1/2 cups Anutra® Cheddar Shreds
1 small head of broccoli, sliced into long thin pieces
1 small head of cauliflower, sliced into long thin pieces
3 medium potatoes, sliced into long thin slices
salt and pepper
vegetable cooking spray

BEAT TOGETHER WELL
1/4 cup Anutra® Cream Cheese
2 cups 99% fat-free egg substitute or egg whites
1/2 cup ANUTRA®
1 cup water
1/2 cup Anutra® Milk

TOPPING - MIX TOGETHER
2 tablespoons Anutra® Parmesan Cheese
2 tablespoons bread crumbs

Heat oil in non-stick skillet, add onions. Sauté until light golden and add mushrooms. Cook another 2 minutes and remove from heat. Heat oven to 375
degrees. Lightly cover a large deep casserole dish with vegetable cooking spray.
Wash vegetables (any combination of those mentioned or whatever you have on
hand). Slice all vegetables into thin slices, the length of each vegetable. Lay
one layer of carrot and zucchini, sprinkle with half of the onions and mushrooms, one-third of the Anutra® Parmesan, lay down a layer of broccoli and
cauliflower, sprinkle with remaining onions and mushrooms, one-third of the
Anutra® Parmesan. Lay down a layer of potatoes. Mix together Anutra®
Milk, Anutra® Cream Cheese and eggs. Pour over mixture. Cover with foil and
bake for 30 minutes. Uncover and bake for 15 minutes. Sprinkle with remaining one-third of the Anutra® Shreds, bread crumbs and Anutra® Parmesan
mixture and bake another 15 minutes.

Nutrition per serving: 317 Calories; 9.1g Fat (26% calories from fat); 21.3g Protein; 40.3g
Carbohydrate; 0mg Cholesterol; 711mg Sodium. Exchanges: 2 Grain (Starch); 2 Lean
Protein; 1-1/2 Vegetable; 1/2 Fat.

BAKED ANUTRA® MACARONI AND CHEESE

Makes 6 Servings

3 cups macaroni
1 tablespoon oil
1 small chopped onion
1 cup sliced mushrooms
1/3 cup ANUTRA®
2/3 cup water
1 cup Anutra® Cheddar Shreds
1/2 cup Anutra® Feta Cheese Crumbles
1/4 teaspoon nutmeg
1/2 teaspoon paprika
salt and pepper — to taste

TOPPING:
1/2 cup bread crumbs
1/2 cup Anutra® Parmesan Cheese
vegetable cooking spray
1/4 cup chopped bell pepper or fresh parsley as garnish

Heat oven to 350 degrees. Boil macaroni for half the required time. (For small shells: about 3 minutes.) Macaroni should still have a definite chew to it, because it will continue to cook in the oven. Set aside. Sauté onions until light golden in color and add mushrooms; sauté another 4 minutes. Stir remaining ingredients together and spoon into a casserole dish sprayed with vegetable cooking spray. Bake for 20 minutes and cover with bread crumb/parmesan mixture. Bake another 10 minutes and garnish with raw green bell pepper or parsley.

Nutrition per serving: 406 Calories; 10.9g Fat (24% calories from fat); 21.4g Protein; 54.6g Carbohydrate; 0mg Cholesterol; 727mg Sodium. Exchanges: 3 Grain (Starch); 2 Lean Protein; 1/2 Vegetable; 1/2 Fat.

BROCCOLI AND ANUTRA® CHEDDAR CASSEROLE

Makes 5 Servings

4 ounces Anutra® Cheddar Shreds — (1 cup)
1 cup cooked long-grain rice
1/2 cup drained canned sliced mushrooms
1/2 cup diced onion
1/4 cup Anutra® Milk
1/4 cup ANUTRA®
1/2 cup water
4 teaspoons Anutra® Butter
1/4 teaspoon salt
20 ounces frozen chopped broccoli — (2 packages) thawed
vegetable cooking spray

Combine the first 9 ingredients in a medium saucepan; cook over low heat 4 minutes or until cheese melts, stirring constantly. Add the broccoli, and cook 2 minutes or until thoroughly heated, stirring frequently. Spoon mixture into a 2-quart casserole coated with cooking spray. Bake at 350 degrees for 30 minutes. Serve.

Nutrition per serving: 181 Calories; 5.9g Fat (29% calories from fat); 11.4g Protein; 23.2g Carbohydrate; 0mg Cholesterol; 593mg Sodium. Exchanges: 1 Grain (Starch); 1 Lean Protein; 1-1/2 Vegetable.

COUSCOUS AND ANUTRA® FETA CRUMBLE CAKES

Makes 8 Servings

2-1/2 cups water
1 cup couscous — uncooked
4 teaspoons olive oil — divided
1 cup minced red onion
1 cup minced red bell pepper
1/2 cup minced green bell pepper
2 garlic cloves — minced
1 cup Anutra® Feta Cheese Crumbles — (4 ounces)
1/2 cup all-purpose flour
1/2 cup ANUTRA®
3/4 cup water
1/2 cup 99% fat-free egg substitute or egg whites
2 tablespoons minced fresh parsley
1/4 teaspoon salt
1/4 teaspoon white pepper

Bring water to a boil in a small saucepan; stir in couscous. Remove from heat; cover and let stand 10 minutes. Fluff with a fork. Place 1 teaspoon oil in a skillet; heat to medium-high. Add onion, bell peppers, and garlic; sauté 5 minutes. Combine couscous, onion mixture, Anutra® Feta Crumbles, and remaining ingredients in a large bowl; stir well. Place 1/2 teaspoon oil in skillet; heat to medium-high heat. Place 1/3 cup couscous mixture for each of 4 portions into skillet, shaping each portion into a 3-inch cake in the skillet. Cook 6 minutes or until golden brown, turning cakes carefully after 3 minutes. Repeat procedure with remaining oil and couscous mixture.

An electric skillet or griddle works well for this recipe because there's more room for the cakes. Otherwise, use a non-stick skillet, and cook in batches. They're delicious plain or served with marinara sauce. Two cakes makes one serving.

Nutrition per serving: 237 Calories; 7.5g Fat (28% calories from fat); 12.3g Protein; 30.2g Carbohydrate; 0mg Cholesterol; 484mg Sodium. Exchanges: 1-1/2 Grain (Starch); 1 Lean Protein; 1/2 Vegetable; 1/2 Fat.

CREAMY ANUTRA® FOUR CHEESE MACARONI

Makes 8 Servings

1/4 cup all-purpose flour
1/2 cup ANUTRA®
1 cup water
1-1/2 cups Anutra® Milk
1-1/2 cups picante sauce
4 Anutra® American Slices
1/2 cup Anutra® Parmesan Cheese
4 ounces Anutra® Cheddar "Chefs Award" — cut in 1/2-inch cubes
4 Anutra® Swiss Slices
6 cups elbow macaroni — cooked
vegetable cooking spray

TOPPING:
2 tablespoons bread crumbs
1 tablespoon Anutra® Parmesan Cheese
vegetable cooking spray

Preheat oven to 375 degrees. Place flour in a large saucepan. Gradually add Anutra® Milk and water stirring with a whisk until blended. Add picante sauce and Anutra®. Cook over medium heat 8 minutes or until thick, stirring constantly. Add cheeses; cook 3 minutes or until cheese melts, stirring frequently. Remove from heat; stir in macaroni. Spoon mixture into a 2-quart casserole coated with cooking spray. Top with bread crumbs and Anutra® Parmesan. Coat lightly with vegetable cooking spray. Bake at 375 degrees for 30 minutes or until bubbly.

Nutrition per serving: 337 Calories; 7.7g Fat (21% calories from fat); 19.6g Protein; 46.3g Carbohydrate; 0mg Cholesterol; 738mg Sodium. Exchanges: 2-1/2 Grain (Starch); 1-1/2 Lean Protein; 1/2 Vegetable; 1/2 Fat.

MAMA LISA'S ANUTRASIZED™
BAKED STUFFED TOMATOES

Makes 2 Servings

2 tomatoes
pinch black pepper
2 tablespoon ANUTRA®
1/4 teaspoon garlic powder
1/4 teaspoon dried basil
1/2 cup Anutra® Shreds - Parmesan, Mozzarella & Romano Blend
1/2 cup bread crumbs
3/4 cup onion — chopped

Heat oven to 375 degrees. Remove stems from tomatoes. Cut in half between blossom end and stem. Squeeze to remove seeds. Slit to the center of the pulp. Season with black pepper, garlic powder, and dried basil. Use fresh chopped garlic and fresh basil if available. Combine Anutra® Shreds, Anutra® and bread crumbs. Fill tomato cavities with mixture. Place stuffed tomatoes on a lightly oiled baking dish with onions. Bake uncovered for 10 minutes and reduce heat to 350 degrees and bake for another 35 minutes. Serve.

Nutrition per serving: 253 Calories; 7.1g Fat (25% calories from fat); 12g Protein; 37.1g Carbohydrate; 0mg Cholesterol; 528mg Sodium. Exchanges: 1-1/2 Grain (Starch); 1 Lean Protein; 2 Vegetable; 1/2 Fat.

MAMA LISA'S ANUTRASIZED™
STUFFED PEPPERS

Makes 2 Servings

2 bell peppers — green, red, or yellow
salt and pepper
2 cups rice, cooked
2 tablespoons ANUTRA®
1/4 cup 99% fat-free egg substitute or egg whites
1/2 cup bread crumbs
1/2 teaspoon garlic powder
1/2 teaspoon dried basil
1/2 cup Anutra® Shreds - Parmesan, Mozzarella & Romano Blend

Cut pepper in half through stem and remove seeds. Sprinkle peppers with a pinch of salt and pepper. Combine cooked rice, egg substitute, bread crumbs, a pinch of salt and pepper, garlic powder, basil and 1/2 cup Anutra® Shreds. Divide mixture in 4 and stuff peppers. Combine remaining bread crumbs and Anutra® Shreds and Anutra®. Place mixture on top of peppers. Bake uncovered for 10 minutes. Reduce heat to 350 degrees and bake for 35 minutes.

Nutrition per serving: 473 Calories; 7.5g Fat (14% calories from fat); 18.4g Protein; 81.7g Carbohydrate; 0mg Cholesterol; 563mg Sodium. Exchanges: 4-1/2 Grain (Starch); 1-1/2 Lean Protein; 1/2 Vegetable; 1/2 Fat.

OPEN FACED ANUTRA® BLUE AND FETA CRUMBLE VEGETABLE SANDWICH

Makes 10 Servings

2 teaspoons olive oil
3 cups onion — cut in 1/2-inch pieces
3 cups mushrooms — diced
1 tablespoon garlic — diced
2 tablespoons balsamic vinegar
2 cups zucchini — diced
2 cups peppers — diced
1 quart stewed tomatoes
1 loaf Italian bread — cut 1-inch thick
1/3 cup ANUTRA®
1/2 cup Anutra® Blue Cheese Crumbles
1/2 cup Anutra® Feta Cheese Crumbles

In hot skillet, add oil. Add onion and mushrooms, sauté until onions are translucent. Add garlic and cook for 1 minute. Add balsamic vinegar and deglaze pan. Add stewed tomatoes, cook at low heat for 5 minutes. Add remaining vegetables. Place bread in toaster or oven until lightly brown. Place bread on a plate and cover each piece of bread with approx 1 cup cooked vegetables. Top vegetables sprinkling with Anutra®, Anutra® Blue and Anutra® Feta Crumbles. Serve.

Nutrition per serving: 267 Calories; 7.3g Fat (25% calories from fat); 12.3g Protein; 40.7g Carbohydrate; 0mg Cholesterol; 761mg Sodium. Exchanges: 1-1/2 Grain (Starch); 1 Lean Protein; 2-1/2 Vegetable; 1/2 Fat.

ORZO AND PORTABELLA ANUTRA®
CASSEROLE

Makes 6 Servings

1/4 cup sun-dried tomatoes — packed without oil
1/4 cup boiling water
1 tablespoon olive oil
2 cups sliced leek
*2 cups diced portabella mushroom caps — *see note*
1 cup quartered mushrooms
2 cloves garlic — minced
4 cups cooked orzo (2 cups uncooked pasta)
1/3 cup ANUTRA®
2/3 cup water
2 cups thinly sliced fennel bulb — 1 large bulb
2 cups low sodium tomato juice
2 tablespoons minced fresh basil
2 tablespoons balsamic vinegar
1 teaspoon paprika
1/8 teaspoon pepper
vegetable cooking spray
1 cup Anutra® Mozzarella Shreds
1/4 cup Anutra® Parmesan Cheese
parsley — optional

Combine the sun-dried tomatoes and boiling water in a small bowl; cover and let stand 10 minutes or until tomatoes soften. Drain. Heat olive oil in large non-stick skillet over medium heat. Add the tomatoes, leek, mushrooms, and garlic; sauté 2 minutes. Combine the mushroom mixture, orzo, and next 8 ingredients (orzo through pepper) in a large bowl; stir well. Spoon mixture into a 13" x 9" baking dish coated with cooking spray. Bake, uncovered, at 400 degrees for 25 minutes. Take out of oven and sprinkle Anutra® Mozzarella Shreds and Anutra® Parmesan over casserole, cover with foil and place back in oven for an additional 7-10 minutes or until shreds have melted. Garnish with parsley sprigs, if desired.

* The portabella mushrooms lend a rich, smoky taste to this dish, but any kind of mushroom can be substituted.

Nutrition per serving: 619.9 Calories; 7.8g Fat (22% calories from fat); 15.1g Protein; 48.6g Carbohydrate; 0mg Cholesterol; 390mg Sodium. Exchanges: 2 Grain (Starch); 1 Lean Protein; 2 Vegetable; 1/2 Fat.

ROASTED TOMATO PASTA FRITTATA WITH ANUTRA® PARMESAN TOAST

Makes 8 Servings

2 garlic cloves — halved
2 tablespoons Anutra® Butter
3 tablespoons Anutra® Parmesan Cheese
1/4 cup ANUTRA®
1 loaf Italian bread — cut into 8 slices
1-1/2 pounds diced tomatoes, peeled, canned
2 tablespoons Anutra® Parmesan Cheese
1/2 teaspoon salt
1/2 teaspoon hot sauce
2 cups 99% fat-free egg substitute or egg whites — lightly beaten
1/2 cup Anutra® Cream Cheese
2 cups cooked spaghetti (5 ounces uncooked pasta)
1 cup basil leaves — torn
2 teaspoons olive oil

Puree garlic, Anutra® Butter, and Anutra® Parmesan Cheese. Rub the mixture on one side of each bread slice, sprinkle with Anutra® and place slices on a baking sheet. Broil 2 minutes or until lightly browned; set Parmesan toast aside. Combine 1 tablespoon Anutra® Parmesan cheese, salt, hot sauce and eggs in a large bowl; stir well. Stir in diced tomato, cooked spaghetti, and basil; set aside. Heat oil in a medium non-stick skillet over low heat. Add egg mixture, and cook 15 minutes or until set (do not stir). Wrap handle of skillet with foil; broil for 3 minutes or until top is set.

Nutrition per serving: 264.8 Calories; 7.3g Fat (25.8% calories from fat); 15.9g Protein; 35g Carbohydrate; 0mg Cholesterol; 702mg Sodium. Exchanges: 1-1/2 Grain (Starch); 1 Lean Protein; 1 Vegetable; 1 Fat.

ROTINI WITH SUN-DRIED TOMATO ANUTRA® BUTTER

Makes 4 Servings

SAUCE:
1/4 sun-dried tomatoes
1/4 cup ANUTRA®
1/2 cup water
1/2 cup Anutra® Butter
1 small shallot — chopped
1-1/2 teaspoons chopped parsley
1/4 teaspoon salt
1/4 teaspoon black pepper

PASTA:
8 ounces rotini
2 tablespoons Anutra® Parmesan Cheese

Cook linguine as directed on box. For sauce, place sun-dried tomatoes in boiling water for one minute (this makes them easier to cut). Rough chop the tomatoes and place in a food processor. Add the rest of the ingredients and blend until smooth. Set aside. When pasta is drained and remains hot, add sun-dried tomato butter. Toss. Top with Anutra® Parmesan. Serve.

Use roasted red peppers instead of sun-dried tomatoes to make roasted red pepper butter sauce. You can use your favorite pasta. Garnish with fresh herbs and vegetables.

Nutrition per serving: 376 Calories; 9.3g Fat (22% calories from fat); 13.8g Protein; 57.3g Carbohydrate; 0mg Cholesterol; 483mg Sodium. Exchanges: 3-1/2 Grain (starch); 1/2 Lean Protein; 1 Fat.

SPINACH AND RISOTTO WITH ANUTRA® ASIAGO AND SUN-DRIED TOMATOES

Makes 6 Servings

4-1/2 cups low sodium vegetable broth
2/3 cup water
2 sun-dried tomatoes — cut in 1/4-inch strips
2 teaspoons olive oil
1/2 cup onion — diced small
1/2 cup celery — diced small
1-1/2 cups uncooked Arborio rice or other short-grain rice
1/3 cup dry white wine
6 cups torn spinach
1/2 cup Anutra® Asiago Cheese Crumbles
1/3 cup ANUTRA®
pinch salt and pepper

Bring broth and water to a simmer in a medium saucepan (do not boil). Combine 1/2 cup warm diluted broth and tomatoes in a bowl; cover and set aside. Keep remaining broth warm over low heat. Heat oil in a large saucepan over medium heat. Add onion; sauté 3 minutes. Add rice; cook 1 minute, stirring constantly. Add wine; cook 1 minute or until liquid is nearly absorbed, stirring constantly. Add warm broth, 1/2 cup at a time, stirring constantly until each portion of broth is absorbed before adding the next (about 20 minutes total). Add tomato mixture and spinach; cook 2 minutes, stirring constantly. Remove from heat; stir in remaining ingredients.

Nutrition per serving: 300 Calories; 4.7g Fat (14% calories from fat); 16.9g Protein; 45.7g Carbohydrate; 0mg Cholesterol; 405mg Sodium. Exchanges: 2-1/2 Grain (Starch); 1-1/2 Lean Protein; 1/2 Vegetable; 1/2 Fat.

SUN-DRIED TOMATO, ANUTRA® FETA AND BASIL RICE CAKES

Makes 8 Servings

3 cups water
1 cup uncooked jasmine or long-grain rice
1/2 cup ANUTRA®
2 cups boiling water
2 ounces sun-dried tomatoes packed without oil and chopped
4 cups eggplant — peeled/diced
pinch of salt
1/2 teaspoon dried Italian seasoning
vegetable cooking spray
1/2 cup finely chopped onion
1 garlic clove — minced
1/2 cup dry bread crumbs
1 cup Anutra® Feta Cheese Crumbles
1/4 cup chopped fresh basil
1/4 cup 99% fat-free egg substitute or egg whites — lightly beaten
2 tablespoons olive oil — divided
basil leaves — optional

Bring 2 cups water to a boil in a medium saucepan. Add rice; cover, reduce heat, and simmer 25 minutes or until liquid is absorbed. Combine 2 cups boiling water and tomatoes in a bowl; let stand 30 minutes or until softened. Drain tomatoes, reserving 1/4 cup liquid. Place eggplant on a foil-lined baking sheet, spreading evenly. Sprinkle salt and Italian seasoning over eggplant. Bake at 375 degrees for 35 minutes or until tender. Heat vegetable cooking spray in a large non-stick skillet over medium-high heat. Add onion and garlic; sauté 3 minutes. Combine onion mixture, rice, Anutra®, remaining water, tomatoes, reserved 1/4 cup liquid, eggplant, bread crumbs, Anutra® Feta Crumbles, basil, and eggs in a large bowl. Divide mixture into 16 equal portions, shaping each into a 3-1/2-inch cake. Heat 1-1/2 teaspoons oil in skillet over medium-high heat. Add 4 cakes, and cook 6 minutes or until golden, turning cakes carefully after 3 minutes. Repeat procedure with remaining oil and cakes.

Serve with Sweet Red Pepper Butter (see recipe page 300), and garnish with basil leaves, if desired.

Nutrition per serving: 266 Calories; 9g Fat (30% calories from fat); 11.7g Protein; 35.1g Carbohydrate; 0mg Cholesterol; 489mg Sodium. Exchanges: 1-1/2 Grain (Starch); 1 Lean Protein; 1/2 Vegetable; 1 Fat.

VEGAN MACARONI AND CHEESE

Makes 10 Servings

3 cups VEGAN CHEESE SAUCE FOR
  MACARONI AND CHEESE (see recipe page 302)
1 quart uncooked macaroni

Cook macaroni according to directions on box. Drain. Prepare Vegan Cheese Sauce and keep warm in sauce pan. Add hot pasta to sauce, stir. Serve.

Nutrition per serving: 285 Calories; 7.5g Fat (24% calories from fat); 11.4g Protein; 41.8g Carbohydrate; 0mg Cholesterol; 958mg Sodium. Exchanges: 2-1/2 Grain (Starch); 1/2 Lean Protein; 1 Fat.

VEGETABLE ANUTRA® CHEESE CASSEROLE

Makes 6 Servings

vegetable cooking spray
12 whole wheat bread slices
1/3 cup ANUTRA®
2/3 cup water
1-1/8 cups Anutra® Shreds - Parmesan, Mozzarella & Romano Blend
1/2 cup chopped green onions
1-1/2 cups 99% fat-free egg substitute or egg whites — slightly beaten
1-1/2 cups Anutra® Milk
1/2 cup Anutra® Cream Cheese
3/4 teaspoon Tabasco® sauce
3/4 teaspoon ground basil
3 tomatoes — thinly sliced
salt and pepper — to taste

Use a 13" x 9" pan or baking dish. Spray pan with vegetable non-stick spray. Place 4 slices of the bread in the bottom of pan and sprinkle Anutra® and with 1/2 cup of the Anutra® Shreds and the green onions. Top with remaining bread slices. Combine eggs, Anutra® Milk, water, Anutra® Cream Cheese, Tabasco®, basil, salt and pepper in small bowl; mix well. Pour the egg mixture over the bread; press so bread is covered with the liquid. Cover and refrigerate 30 minutes or longer. Uncover and top with thin slices of tomatoes and sprinkle with the remaining cheese. Bake in preheated 350 degree oven 30-35 minutes. It is done when a knife inserted near center comes out clean. Let stand 10-15 minutes before serving.

Nutrition per serving: 284 Calories; 9g Fat (29% calories from fat); 20.8g Protein; 32.7g Carbohydrate; 0mg Cholesterol; 824mg Sodium. Exchanges: 1-1/2 Grain (Starch); 2 Lean Protein; 1/2 Fat.

ANUTRA® BLUE CHEESE AND WALNUT RISOTTO

Makes 5 Servings

2 cups low sodium vegetable broth
1/2 cup water
1/4 cup ANUTRA®
1 teaspoon olive oil
1/3 cup onion — diced small
1/3 cup celery — diced small
3/4 cup uncooked Arborio rice or other short-grain rice
3 tablespoons dry white wine
1/4 cup walnuts — chopped
1/3 cup Anutra® Blue Cheese Crumbles
2 tablespoons Anutra® Parmesan Cheese
pinch salt and pepper

Bring broth and water to a simmer in a medium saucepan (do not boil). Keep remaining broth warm over low heat. Heat oil in a large saucepan over medium heat. Add onion and celery; sauté 3 minutes. Add rice and Anutra®; cook 1 minute, stirring constantly. Add wine; cook 1 minute or until liquid is nearly absorbed, stirring constantly. Add warm diluted broth, 1/2 cup at a time, stirring constantly until each portion of broth is absorbed before adding the next (about 20 minutes total). Remove from heat, stir in remaining ingredients.

Nutrition per serving: 245 Calories; 8.4g Fat (31% calories from fat); 13.6g Protein; 28.2g Carbohydrate; 0mg Cholesterol; 377mg Sodium. Exchanges: 1-1/2 Grain (Starch); 1-1/2 Lean Protein; 1 Fat.

ANUTRA® BURRITOS CON QUESOS

Makes 8 Servings

1/2 tablespoon olive oil
3 yellow onions — sliced thin
1 large bell pepper — julienned
1 jalapeño pepper — chopped
15 ounces tomatoes, canned — peeled and chopped
2 cups 99% fat-free egg substitute or egg whites
1/2 cup ANUTRA®
2 cups Anutra® Cheddar Shreds
8 flour tortillas

Cut the onions into thin slices and separate the slices into individual rings. Julienne the green pepper. Mince the jalapeño pepper (use a canned one if necessary). In a large heavy skillet, heat 1/2 tablespoon oil; add the onions and green peppers. Sauté until onions are translucent and limp. Add the chopped tomato and the minced jalapeño and continue cooking for 3 minutes more. Add the eggs which have been lightly beaten, Anutra® and water and blend well. Add Anutra® Cheddar Shreds to egg mixture and pour in skillet. Proceed as though you were scrambling eggs. Warm the flour tortillas while cooking the filling, or quickly run each tortilla over the flame on a gas stove, just to soften. Fill each tortilla with 1/8th of the mixture. Roll the tortillas by turning one side up and folding the edges inward. Wrap the lower third in foil or waxed paper and serve immediately.

You can also serve with Anutra® Sour Cream and avocado.

Nutrition per serving: 264 Calories; 8.5g Fat (29% calories from fat); 15.9g Protein; 31.3g Carbohydrate; 0mg Cholesterol; 731mg Sodium. Exchanges: 1-1/2 Grain (Starch); 1-1/2 Lean Protein; 1-1/2 Vegetable; 1/2 Fat.

ANUTRA® CHEDDAR EGG FRIED RICE

Makes 5 Servings

2 teaspoons dark sesame oil
1 cup 99% fat-free egg substitute or egg whites
1 tablespoon vegetable oil
4 cups cooked rice — cold
5 tablespoons ANUTRA®
1 cup frozen green peas — thawed
1/4 teaspoon salt
1/4 teaspoon pepper
1 cup bean sprouts
1/3 cup chopped green onions
5 Anutra® Cheddar Slices — cut in 1/2-inch strips

Combine the sesame oil and eggs in a small bowl; stir well, and set aside. Heat vegetable oil in a large non-stick skillet or wok over medium-high heat. Add egg mixture, and stir-fry 2 minutes. Add rice; stir-fry 3 minutes. Add green peas, salt, and pepper; stir-fry 5 minutes. Add bean sprouts, green onion, and Anutra® Slices. Stir-fry 1-2 minutes until cheese melts. Sprinkle with Anutra®. Serve immediately.

Nutrition per serving: 354 Calories; 9.1g Fat (23% calories from fat); 15.1g Protein; 51.9g Carbohydrate; 0mg Cholesterol; 474mg Sodium. Exchanges: 3 Grain (Starch); 1 Lean Protein; 1/2 Vegetable; 1-1/2 Fat.

ANUTRA® CHEESE BREAD PUDDING

Makes 4 Servings

8 slices stale bread — cubed
1 cup Anutra® Cheddar Shreds
1-1/2 cups Anutra® Milk
1/2 cup water
3/4 cup 99% fat-free egg substitute or egg whites
1/4 cup ANUTRA®
3 tablespoons Anutra® Cream Cheese
2 teaspoons Dijon mustard
1/4 teaspoon cayenne pepper
1/2 teaspoon Worcestershire sauce

Spray a 1-quart baking dish with vegetable cooking spray. Layer half the bread cubes in the dish. Sprinkle with half the cheese. Repeat with remaining bread cubes and cheese. Beat remaining ingredients together and pour over bread and cheese. Let stand one hour. Place baking dish in a 9" x 13" pan and pour water into pan to a depth of one inch. Place pan in preheated 350 degree oven and bake one hour. Pudding should be puffy and golden.

Nutrition per serving: 302 Calories; 9g Fat (27% calories from fat); 20.1g Protein; 35.4g Carbohydrate; 0mg Cholesterol; 891mg Sodium. Exchanges: 2 Grain (Starch); 2 Lean Protein; 1/2 Fat.

ANUTRA® CHEESY MEATLESS BURRITO

Makes 2 Servings

1/2 cup onion — diced
2 vegetable burger patties— crumbled
1/2 cup diced tomatoes, peeled, canned
1/2 teaspoon cumin
1/2 teaspoon oregano
1/2 teaspoon garlic powder
1/4 cup Anutra® Shreds - Monterey Jack and Cheddar Blend
2 tablespoons ANUTRA®
2 flour tortillas
1/2 cup shredded lettuce

Heat cooking skillet to medium high heat. Add oil. Add onion and let cook for about 1 minute. Add next 5 ingredients and let cook for 4-5 minutes for flavors to blend. Take off heat and fold in Anutra® Shreds and Anutra®. Put tortilla in microwave oven for approx 1 minute or until soft. Place mixture across tortilla in middle. Place shredded lettuce on top of filling. Fold left and right sides approx 1 inch and wrap. Serve with salsa and Anutra® Sour Cream.

Nutrition per serving: 336 Calories; 11.2g Fat (30% calories from fat); 23.5g Protein; 35.4g Carbohydrate; 0mg Cholesterol; 628mg Sodium. Exchanges: 1-1/2 Grain (Starch); 2-1/2 Lean Protein; 1 Vegetable; 2 Fat.

ANUTRA® CHEESY PASTA CARBONARA

Makes 6 Servings

6 ounces bacon, meatless — chopped
2 cloves garlic — minced
6 cups hot cooked thin spaghetti
1-1/2 cups uncooked pasta
1/4 cup Anutra® Parmesan Cheese
1 cup Anutra® Shreds - Monterey Jack and Cheddar Blend
2 tablespoons minced fresh parsley
1/4 teaspoon freshly ground pepper
1/2 cup Anutra® Milk
1/3 cup ANUTRA®
2/3 cup water
1 tablespoon Anutra® Cream Cheese
1/2 cup egg substitute

Cook meatless bacon in a large non-stick skillet over medium-high heat until crisp. Add garlic and sauté 1 minute or until tender. Reduce heat to low; stir in pasta, Anutra® Parmesan and Monterey Jack Shreds, parsley, and pepper. Combine Anutra® Milk, water, Anutra®, Anutra® Cream Cheese, and eggs; stir well. Pour mixture over pasta mixture, and cook 3 minutes or until sauce thickens, stirring constantly. Serve immediately.

Nutrition per serving: 416 Calories; 16.5g Fat (36% calories from fat); 20.3g Protein; 47.7g Carbohydrate; 0mg Cholesterol; 827mg Sodium. Exchanges: 2-1/2 Grain (Starch); 2 Lean Protein; 1-1/2 Fat.

ANUTRA® FETA AND VEGETABLE LASAGNA

Makes 8 Servings

ANUTRA® FETA FILLING:
15 ounces Anutra® Feta Cheese
  Crumbles
1 tablespoon fresh parsley —
  chopped fine
1 teaspoon chives — chopped
1 tablespoon fresh basil leaf —
  chopped
1 teaspoon garlic powder
1 teaspoon onion powder
1/4 teaspoon thyme
1/4 cup Anutra® Mozzarella Shreds
1/2 teaspoon oregano
2 tablespoons Anutra® Garlic Herb
  Parmesan
1/2 cup ANUTRA®
1 cup water

SPINACH FILLING:
1 teaspoon olive oil
9 ounces frozen chopped spinach
1 teaspoon garlic — chopped
1/3 cup diced onion

LASAGNA:
1-1/3 cups low sodium marinara
  sauce
8 oven ready lasagna noodles —
  (do not preboil)
1 zucchini - cut lengthwise 1/4-inch
2 yellow squash - cut lengthwise
  1/4-inch
1 cup mushrooms — thinly sliced
1/2 cup Anutra® Mozzarella Shreds
vegetable cooking spray

For the feta filling, place all ingredients in food processor and mix
well.

For spinach filling, squeeze out as much water as you can from
spinach. Set aside. In a sauté pan, heat oil, add garlic and spinach.
Sauté until dry. Cool until ready to use.

Preheat oven to 400 degrees. Assemble lasagna in an 8" x 8" x 2"
Pyrex pan lightly coated with vegetable cooking spray. Build
lasagna in this order: Spread 1/3 cup of marinara sauce on bottom,
2 oven ready lasagna noodles, 1 layer of zucchini, 1 layer of yellow
squash, 1/4 cup marinara sauce, 1 cup of Anutra® Feta filling,
mushrooms, yellow squash, 1/4 cup marinara sauce, Anutra® Feta
filling, 1/2 cup Anutra® Mozzarella, 3 oven ready lasagna noodles,
1/2 cup marinara sauce and top with 1 cup Anutra® Mozzarella
Shreds. Cover with foil and bake 1 hour.

Nutrition per serving: 536 Calories; 11.5g Fat (19% calories from fat); 28.9g
Protein; 79.7g Carbohydrate; 0mg Cholesterol; 750mg Sodium. Exchanges: 4-1/2
Grain (Starch); 2-1/2 Lean Protein; 1-1/2 Vegetable.

ANUTRA® FOUR CHEESE ROASTED VEGETABLE LASAGNA

Makes 10 Servings

1-1/2 teaspoons olive oil
1 teaspoon garlic powder
1 onion — cut 1/2-inch thick
2 zucchinis, whole — cut 1/2-inch thick
1 cup mushrooms — sliced
1 each red and green bell pepper — cut 1/2-inch thick
2 cups diced tomato — drained
3-1/2 cups marinara sauce — your favorite
2/3 cup ANUTRA®
1-1/3 cup water

1 teaspoon oregano
1 teaspoon basil
1 cup Anutra® Mozzarella Shreds
1 cup Anutra® Shreds - Parmesan, Mozzarella & Romano Blend
1/2 cup Anutra® Feta Cheese Crumbles
1/2 cup Anutra® Parmesan Cheese
9 oven ready lasagna noodles — (do not preboil)
2 tablespoons fresh parsley — chopped fine

Preheat oven to 400 degrees. Place all vegetables in a large bowl. Toss with herbs and olive oil. Place on roasting pan and roast for 30 minutes. Drain off excess liquid. Divide in half. Set aside. Toss all Anutra® Cheeses in bowl. Set aside. Assemble in an 13" x 9" x 2" baking pan-following these steps:
   Lightly coat pan with non stick spray
   2/3 cup marinara sauce
   3 oven ready lasagna noodles
   2/3 cup marinara sauce
   1/2 all roasted vegetables
   1 cup Anutra® Cheese mixture
   3 oven ready lasagna noodles
   2/3 cup marinara sauce (pre-mixed with Anutra® and water)
   2nd half roasted vegetables
   1 cup Anutra® Cheese mixture
   3 oven ready noodles
   1 cup marinara sauce
Cover with foil and bake 45 minutes. Take out of oven. Place 1/2 cup of marinara sauce on top and 1 cup of Anutra® Cheese Mixture. Sprinkle with 1 teaspoon dried basil. Recover with foil and place back in oven for 10 minutes. Take out of oven; sprinkle with fresh parsley. Let set for 10-15 minutes. Serve.

Nutrition per serving: 230 Calories; 7g Fat (27% calories from fat); 13.2g Protein; 31g Carbohydrate; 0mg Cholesterol; 589mg Sodium. Exchanges: 1 Grain (Starch); 1 Lean Protein; 2-1/2 Vegetable.

ANUTRA® FOUR-CHEESE MANICOTTI

Makes 6 Servings

12 Manicotti — uncooked
vegetable cooking spray
1/2 cup finely chopped onion
3 garlic cloves — minced
1 cup Anutra® Mozzarella Shreds — divided
1/2 cup Anutra® Parmesan Cheese — divided
1 teaspoon dried Italian seasoning
1/2 teaspoon pepper
1/2 cup Anutra® Asiago Cheese Crumbles
1/2 cup Anutra® Cream Cheese — softened
1/2 package frozen chopped spinach — 10-ounce,
*   thawed, drained, and squeezed dry*
27-1/2 ounces low sodium marinara sauce — optional
6 tablespoons ANUTRA®

Cook pasta according to package directions, omitting salt; set aside.
Coat a small non-stick skillet with cooking spray, and place over
medium-high heat until hot. Add onion and garlic; sauté 3 minutes.
Remove from heat; set aside. Combine 1/2 cup Anutra®
Mozzarella Shreds, 1/4 cup Anutra® Parmesan, and next 4 ingredients in a bowl; beat with a mixer at medium speed until smooth.
Stir in onion mixture and spinach. Spoon mozzarella mixture into
cooked manicotti (about 1/3 cup per shell). Divide 1 cup sauce
evenly between 6 individual casserole dishes coated with cooking
spray. Arrange 2 stuffed manicotti in each dish. Pour remaining
sauce over each serving. Place dishes on a baking sheet. Cover
each dish with foil, and bake at 350 degrees for 25 minutes.
Sprinkle with remaining Anutra® Mozzarella and Parmesan; bake,
uncovered, an additional 5 minutes. Sprinkle each with 1 tablespoon of Anutra® Garnish with oregano, if desired.

If you don't have individual casserole dishes, use a 13" x 9" baking
dish to prepare this entrée.

Nutrition per serving: 370 Calories; 9.9g Fat (24% calories from fat); 22.5g
Protein; 51g Carbohydrate; 0mg Cholesterol; 816mg Sodium. Exchanges: 2 Lean
Protein; 3 Vegetable; 1/2 Fat.

ANUTRA® GARLIC AND HERBED PARMESAN ORZO

Makes 6 Servings

1/2 cup onion — diced small
1/2 cup celery — diced small
1-1/2 cups Vegan Cheddar Cheese Sauce Alternative
3 cups orzo — dry
1/4 cup Anutra® Garlic Herb Parmesan
6 tablespoons ANUTRA®

Cook orzo as directed on box. Set aside. Heat medium sauce pan to medium high heat and add vegetable non-stick spray. Add onion and celery cooking for approx 1 minute stirring as needed. Add Vegan Cheese Sauce, orzo, and Anutra® Parmesan Cheese. Heat to simmer and cook for 5 minutes. Serve Sprinkle with Anutra®.

Nutrition per serving: 285 Calories; 7.2g Fat (23% calories from fat); 12.6g Protein; 41.4g Carbohydrate; 0mg Cholesterol; 872mg Sodium. Exchanges: 2-1/2 Grain (Starch); 1/2 Lean Protein; 1/2 Vegetable; 1 Fat.

ANUTRA® ITALIAN BEANS AND RICE

Makes 4 Servings

1/2 cup navy beans — dried
2 cups water
2 tablespoons olive oil
1 medium onion — chopped
1 small clove garlic — minced
3/4 cup chopped celery
1-1/2 cups canned tomatoes — undrained or peeled fresh tomatoes
2 cups low sodium vegetable broth
1/8 teaspoon cayenne pepper
1 teaspoon oregano
1/4 teaspoon thyme
1/2 cup rice
3/4 cup Anutra® Shreds - Parmesan, Mozzarella & Romano Blend
1/2 tablespoon Anutra® Parmesan Cheese
4 tablespoons ANUTRA®
salt and pepper — to taste

Cover beans with water and bring to a boil for 2 minutes, remove from heat and soak for an hour. Then cook for approx one hour until tender on simmer heat. When necessary, add more vegetable broth as the beans are cooking. Sauté the onion and garlic in the olive oil until light golden in color, add the celery and stir this mixture into the beans. Add tomatoes, cayenne, herbs, and enough water or chicken stock to cover the mixture. Add rice, cover and simmer stirring about every 5 minutes for 20 minutes, or until the rice is cooked. Fold in Anutra® Shreds and spoon into bowls. Top with Anutra® Parmesan and Anutra®.

You can skip the bean cooking step by using canned beans. Take canned beans, drain, and add to onion and garlic after they are sautéed. Continue with the recipe.

Nutrition per serving: 369 Calories; 11.9g Fat (29% calories from fat); 20.4g Protein; 47.2g Carbohydrate; 0mg Cholesterol; 664mg Sodium. Exchanges: 2-1/2 Grain (Starch); 2 Lean Protein; 1-1/2 Vegetable; 1-1/2 Fat.

ANUTRA® MONTEREY AND CHEDDAR RISOTTO CASSEROLE

Makes 8 Servings

1 tablespoon olive oil
1/2 cup onion — diced
1/2 cup celery — diced
1 cup risotto — uncooked
1/2 cup ANUTRA®
3-1/2 cups low sodium vegetable broth
1 cup water
2 cups Anutra® Shreds - Monterey Jack and Cheddar Blend
20 ounce package of frozen chopped broccoli — thawed and drained
1/8 teaspoon cayenne pepper
1/2 tablespoon basil
1/2 teaspoon thyme
2 teaspoons garlic powder
1/2 cup almond slivers
vegetable cooking spray

Preheat oven to 375 degrees. Heat medium sized sauce pan to medium-high heat, add oil, onion and celery. Sauté for 3 minutes. Add risotto and stir until risotto is well coated with oil. Add diluted vegetable stock in thirds incorporating as risotto and Anutra® absorbs liquids, stirring occasionally. Once stock has all been added, fold in Anutra® Shreds, Anutra® Parmesan, broccoli, herbs and spices, and almonds. Place mixture in a lightly sprayed 2 quart baking dish. Bake for 30 minutes.

Nutrition per serving: 277 Calories; 10.9g Fat (35% calories from fat); 17.3g Protein; 29.9g Carbohydrate; 0mg Cholesterol; 535mg Sodium. Exchanges: 1-1/2 Grain (Starch); 1 Lean Protein; 1 Vegetable; 1 Fat.

ANUTRA® MOZZARELLA EGGPLANT PARMESAN

Makes 8 Servings

3 cups low sodium marinara sauce
28 ounces canned tomatoes, drained and chopped
2 garlic cloves — minced
1 pound eggplant, slice crosswise 1/4-inch
1-1/4 cup water
1/2 cup ANUTRA®
3 egg whites — lightly beaten
1 cup bread crumbs — Italian seasoned
1/4 cup Anutra® Parmesan Cheese
vegetable cooking spray
2 cups Anutra® Mozzarella Shreds
fresh oregano sprigs — optional

Combine first 8 ingredients in a large saucepan; bring to a boil.
Reduce heat and simmer, uncovered, 20 minutes. Place eggplant in
a large bowl; add water to cover, and let stand 30 minutes. Drain
well; blot dry with paper towels. Combine 1/4 cup water and eggs in
a shallow bowl. Combine bread crumbs and parmesan cheese; stir
well. Dip eggplant in egg mixture, and dredge in bread crumb mixture. Place half of eggplant on a baking sheet coated with cooking
spray, and broil 5 minutes on each side or until browned. Repeat
procedure with remaining eggplant. Set eggplant aside. Spread
half of tomato mixture in bottom of a 13" x 9" baking dish coated
with cooking spray. Arrange half of eggplant over sauce; top with
half of mozzarella shreds. Repeat layers with remaining sauce, eggplant, and shreds. Bake at 350 degrees for 30 minutes or until bubbly. Let stand 5 minutes before serving. Garnish with fresh parsley.

Nutrition per serving: 237.4 Calories; 7.3g Fat (28.9% calories from fat); 14.4g
Protein; 31.3g Carbohydrate; 0mg Cholesterol; 750mg Sodium. Exchanges: 1/2
Grain (Starch); 1-1/2 Lean Protein; 3 Vegetable.

ANUTRA® MUSHROOM STROGANOFF

Makes 8 Servings

1 tablespoon olive oil
8 ounces onion — pearl
1 tablespoon garlic — minced
8 ounces mushrooms — cut in 1/2-inch slices
6 ounces portabella mushrooms — cut in 1/2-inch slices
1 cup low sodium vegetable broth
3/4 cup Anutra® Cream Cheese
1/4 cup low sodium vegetable broth
1 cup water
1/2 cup ANUTRA®
2 teaspoons cornstarch
2 tablespoons cooking sherry
pinch salt and pepper
4 cups spinach noodles, cooked

Heat medium non-stick stock pot to medium-high heat. Add olive oil, onion, let cook for 5 minutes. Onions should caramelize on outside. Add mushrooms and cook for 7 minutes. Slowly add stock to pan continuing to incorporate flavors from the mushrooms and onions. Take pan off the heat and strain vegetables. Let broth cool until warm and whisk in Anutra® Cream Cheese until well combined. Combine 1/4 cup vegetable stock, 1 cup water, and Anutra® with 2 teaspoons of cornstarch. Add stock back to pan, slowly add cornstarch mixture and cook on medium heat until sauce has thickened. Add cooking sherry and season to taste. Serve on top of spinach noodles.

Nutrition per serving: 417 Calories; 12.7g Fat (27% calories from fat); 23.6g Protein; 56.2g Carbohydrate; 0mg Cholesterol; 511mg Sodium. Exchanges: 2-1/2 Grain (Starch); 1 Lean Protein; 2 Vegetable; 2 Fat.

ANUTRA® PARMESAN AND BLUE CHEESE ORZO

Makes 2 Servings

1 tablespoon Anutra® Parmesan Cheese
2 tablespoons Anutra® Cream Cheese
2 tablespoons Anutra® Blue Cheese Crumbles
2 tablespoons ANUTRA®
2 tablespoons Anutra® Milk
4 tablespoons water
1/8 teaspoon salt
1/8 teaspoon pepper
2 tablespoons roasted red peppers — diced
2/3 cup orzo — (rice-shaped pasta)
1/3 cup sliced green onions

Combine first 7 ingredients in a bowl; beat with an electric mixer at medium speed until smooth. Stir in roasted red peppers. Cook orzo in boiling water 8 minutes. Add green onions and cook an additional 2 minutes; drain well. Add to Anutra® mixture; stir well. Serve immediately.

Nutrition per serving: 211 Calories; 6g Fat (26% calories from fat); 12.5g Protein; 27.8g Carbohydrate; 0mg Cholesterol; 511mg Sodium. Exchanges: 1-1/2 Grain (Starch); 1 Lean Protein; 1/2 Vegetable; 1/2 Fat.

ANUTRA® PARMESAN CREPES

Makes 12 Servings

1-1/4 cups all-purpose flour
1/4 cup Anutra® Parmesan Cheese
1-1/2 cups Anutra® Milk
1 tablespoon Anutra® Butter — melted
1 teaspoon olive oil
1/4 cup 99% fat-free egg substitute or egg whites
vegetable cooking spray

Place flour in a medium bowl. Combine Anutra® Milk, Anutra® Butter, and eggs, and add mixture to flour, stirring with a wire whisk until almost smooth. Cover batter and chill for 1 hour.

Coat an 8-inch-crepe pan or non-stick skillet with vegetable cooking spray, and place over medium-high heat until hot. Remove pan from heat, and pour a scant 1/4 cup batter into pan; quickly tilt pan in all directions so batter covers pan with a thin film. Cook about 1 minute.

Carefully lift edge of crepe with spatula to test for doneness. The crepe is ready to turn when it can be shaken loose from pan and the underside is lightly browned. Turn crepe over, and cook 30 seconds on the other side. Place the crepe on a towel and allow it to cool. Repeat procedure until all of the batter is used. Stack crepes between single layers of wax paper or paper towels to prevent sticking.

Fill these crepes with beans, eggs, one tablespoon of Anutra® or your favorite vegetables. Cooled crepes can be stacked in wax paper and frozen in a zip-lock bag for up to three months.

Nutrition per serving: 104 Calories; 3.3g Fat (29% calories from fat); 4.9g Protein; 14.1g Carbohydrate; 0mg Cholesterol; 74mg Sodium. Exchanges: 1 Grain (Starch); 1/2 Lean Protein.

ANUTRA® PASTA PUTTANESCA

Makes 6 Servings

2 onions — diced
2 tablespoons olive oil
4 garlic cloves — minced
28 ounces canned whole plum tomatoes — drained and diced
2 black olives — pitted and halved
1 teaspoon hot-pepper flakes
1 teaspoon dried oregano
1 teaspoon dried basil
1/4 teaspoon fresh ground pepper
12 ounces dried fusilli or other dried pasta
1/2 cup Anutra® Asiago Cheese Crumbles
1/3 cup ANUTRA®

In a medium saucepan or large skillet over medium heat, sauté onions in oil until translucent (about 4 minutes). Add garlic and cook 3 minutes. Stir in tomatoes, olives, hot-pepper flakes, oregano, basil, and pepper; reduce heat to medium-low and simmer 15 minutes. In a large saucepan, bring 4 quarts water to a boil. Cook pasta as directed on box. Serve immediately. Sprinkle with Anutra® Asiago Cheese Crumbles and Anutra®.

This can also be made with additions of navy beans, or fresh seasonal produce such as asparagus, broccoli, or bell peppers.

Nutrition per serving: 368 Calories; 10.7g Fat (26% calories from fat); 12.5g Protein; 57.3g Carbohydrate; 0mg Cholesterol; 572mg Sodium. Exchanges: 3 Grain (Starch); 1/2 Lean Protein; 2 Vegetable; 1-1/2 Fat.

ANUTRA® ROMAINE FRITTATA

Makes 2 Servings

2 tablespoons Anutra® Butter
1 cup romaine lettuce — coarsely chopped
1 cup 99% fat-free egg substitute or egg whites
2 tablespoons ANUTRA®
1 pinch sea salt
1 pinch fresh ground black pepper
1/4 cup Anutra® Shreds - Parmesan, Mozzarella & Romano Blend

Preheat broiler at a full broil. Heat sauté pan or skillet; spray with non-stick spray, add lettuce and cook, stirring for 2 minutes. Beat eggs with Anutra® Butter and Anutra® in a small bowl until fluffy; add seasoning to taste and pour over lettuce. Let cook gently over medium heat until set on bottom, about 2 minutes.

Sprinkle grated cheese over top. Put pan under preheated broiler until cheese melts and top puffs, about 1 minute. Take pan to table and serve hot.

Nutrition per serving: 152 Calories; 6.6g Fat (39% calories from fat); 15g Protein; 7.6g Carbohydrate; 0mg Cholesterol; 546mg Sodium. Exchanges: 1/2 Grain (Starch); 2 Lean Protein; 1/2 Fat.

ANUTRA® SOUTHWEST TORTA

Makes 8 Servings

vegetable cooking spray
7 flour tortillas (10-inch diameter)
1 pound vegetable burger —
  crumbled
1 onion — diced
1 red bell pepper — diced
1 jalapeño — diced
1 teaspoon chili powder
1/4 teaspoon dried oregano
1 tablespoon cumin
15 ounces cooked black beans

3/4 cup Anutra® Shreds - Monterey
  Jack and Cheddar Blend
2 cups 99% fat-free egg substitute
  or egg whites — beaten
1/2 cup ANUTRA®
1/2 cup water
1/4 cup Anutra® Cream Cheese
1/4 teaspoon fresh ground black
  pepper
3 green onions — diced

Preheat oven to 350 degrees. Line a 9-inch springform pan with aluminum foil. Spray foil with vegetable cooking spray. Place 5 tortillas around perimeter of foil-lined pan. Place 1 tortilla in center of pan to cover bottom entirely. Spray tortillas with vegetable cooking spray. In a large skillet over medium heat, cook vegetable burger until browned and crumbly (about 10 minutes). Add onion, bell pepper, chile, chili powder, oregano, and cumin and cook until onion is tender (about 10 minutes). Place vegetable burger mixture in tortilla-lined baking dish; reserve cooking pan. Cover mixture with beans and Anutra® Shreds. In a medium sized bowl, beat egg substitute, Anutra®, water and Anutra® Cream Cheese. In reserved skillet over medium heat, apply vegetable cooking spray and scramble egg substitute. Stir in pepper and green onions, undercooking eggs slightly. Press eggs over beans and Anutra® Cheese. Place remaining tortilla over eggs. Lightly coat with vegetable cooking spray. Place in oven and bake 25 minutes. Cool 5 minutes before serving. To unmold, loosen edge with a knife; remove pan sides. Loosen pan bottom then remove. Peel away foil. Cut torta into 8 wedges and serve.

If it is more convenient, prepare this colorful and simple torta ahead and warm in a 350 degree oven for 20 minutes before serving.

Nutrition per serving: 422 Calories; 12.8g Fat (27% calories from fat); 31.6g Protein; 45.7g Carbohydrate; 0mg Cholesterol; 618mg Sodium. Exchanges: 2 Grain (Starch); 3-1/2 Lean Protein; 1 Vegetable; 2-1/2 Fat.

ANUTRA® VEGETABLE AND BLACK BEAN SOFT TACOS

Makes 6 Servings

1 tablespoon olive oil
2 cups coarsely chopped broccoli florets — 1/2 bunch
1 cup sliced red onion
1 cup julienne-cut green bell pepper
1/2 cup julienne-cut red bell pepper
1 cup sliced mushrooms
1 cup sliced shiitake mushroom caps
1/3 cup minced seeded Anaheim chile
1/2 teaspoon ground cumin
1/2 teaspoon chili powder
1/2 cup tomato juice
1/3 cup ANUTRA®
2/3 cup water
1 tablespoon minced fresh cilantro
2 tablespoons fresh lime juice
15 ounces canned black beans — drained and rinsed
6 flour tortillas — 10-inch diameter
1-1/2 cups Anutra® Shreds - Monterey Jack and Cheddar Blend
3 cups thinly sliced iceberg lettuce
3/4 cup medium salsa
6 tablespoons Anutra® Sour Cream

Heat oil in a large non-stick skillet over medium-high heat. Add broccoli, onion, and bell peppers; sauté 4 minutes. Add mushrooms, chile, cumin, and chili powder; sauté 2 minutes. Add tomato juice, Anutra® and water; cook 2 minutes or until slightly thickened. Remove from heat; stir in minced cilantro and lime juice and set aside. Divide black beans evenly among tortillas; top each with 1/2 cup broccoli mixture and 1/4 cup Anutra® Shreds. Fold tortillas in half, and place on a baking sheet. Bake at 375 degrees for 5 minutes or until cheese melts. Serve with lettuce, salsa, and Anutra® Sour Cream.

Nutrition per serving: 385 Calories; 12.2g Fat (29% calories from fat); 19.7g Protein; 52.9g Carbohydrate; 0mg Cholesterol; 752mg Sodium. Exchanges: 2-1/2 Grain (Starch); 1-1/2 Lean Protein; 2 Vegetable; 1 Fat.

ANUTRA® ZITI

Makes 4 Servings

2 cups ziti pasta — dry
1 teaspoon olive oil
1 tablespoon olive oil
1/2 each red and green bell peppers — chopped
1 onion — chopped
6 button mushrooms
2 garlic cloves — minced
1 teaspoon dried oregano
1/2 teaspoon dried thyme
2 cups crushed tomatoes, low sodium — canned
4 tablespoons ANUTRA®
1/2 cup water
pinch salt and pepper
1-1/2 cups Anutra® Mozzarella Shreds

Preheat oven to 375 degrees. Cook pasta according to directions on package. Drain and return to pot. Toss with 1 teaspoon of olive oil. Heat remaining olive oil in 2 tablespoons in a large skillet over medium heat. Add bell pepper, onion, mushrooms, garlic, oregano, and thyme. Cook for 5 minutes, stirring occasionally. Add salt and pepper. Stir in crushed tomatoes, Anutra®, water and cook 5 minutes. Add pasta and 1 cup of Anutra® Mozzarella Shreds tossing to combine. Pour into lightly sprayed 3 quart shallow baking dish, top with remaining shreds. Bake for 20-25 minutes or until slightly brown.

Nutrition per serving: 421 Calories; 12.6g Fat (27% calories from fat); 20.5g Protein; 59.2g Carbohydrate; 0mg Cholesterol; 580mg Sodium. Exchanges: 2-1/2 Grain (Starch); 1-1/2 Lean Protein; 3 Vegetable; 1 Fat.

ZUCCHINI AND ANUTRA® MOZZARELLA CHEESE CASSEROLE

Makes 4 Servings

4 ounces spaghetti — broken
1/2 tablespoon olive oil
2/3 cup chopped onions
1 cup chopped green bell peppers
1-1/2 pounds sliced zucchini
4 fresh tomatoes — cut in wedges
1/4 cup chopped parsley
1/8 teaspoon black pepper
1-1/2 cups Anutra® Mozzarella Shreds
4 tablespoons ANUTRA®

Preheat oven to 350 degrees. Cook spaghetti as directed on box; drain; cool; set aside. Sauté onion for 2 minutes in olive oil; add green pepper, zucchini, tomatoes, parsley and pepper. Cook about 5 minutes. Lightly coat casserole dish with vegetable cooking spray, add spaghetti and zucchini mixture. Sprinkle Anutra® Mozzarella and Anutra® on top; cover and bake for 20 minutes. Remove cover and cook another 5 minutes until hot and bubbly. Garnish with fresh chopped parsley.

Nutrition per serving: 305 Calories; 9.4g Fat (28% calories from fat); 17.3g Protein; 41g Carbohydrate; 0mg Cholesterol; 607mg Sodium. Exchanges: 1-1/2 Grain 9starch); 1-1/2 Lean Protein; 2-1/2 Vegetable; 1/2 Fat.

MY FAVORITE ENTRÉE - ANUTRASIZED™:

Makes _____Servings

Ingredients:

_____   _____
_____   _____
_____   _____
_____   _____
_____   _____
_____   _____
_____   _____

Instructions:

_____
_____
_____
_____
_____
_____
_____
_____
_____
_____
_____
_____
_____
_____
_____

Nutrition per serving:
_____Calories;   _____g Fat (_____% Fat Cal);   _____g Protein;
_____g Carbohydrate;   _____mg Cholesterol;   _____mg Sodium.
Exchanges:
_____Grain (Starch);   _____Lean Protein;   _____Vegetable;
_____Fruit;   _____Other Carbohydrate

MY 2ND FAVORITE ENTRÉE - ANUTRASIZED™:

Makes _____ Servings

Ingredients:

_____   _____
_____   _____
_____   _____
_____   _____
_____   _____
_____   _____

Instructions:

_____
_____
_____
_____
_____
_____
_____
_____
_____
_____
_____
_____
_____
_____

Nutrition per serving:
_____Calories;   _____g Fat (_____% Fat Cal);   _____g Protein;
_____g Carbohydrate;   _____mg Cholesterol;   _____mg Sodium.
Exchanges:
_____Grain (Starch);   _____Lean Protein;   _____Vegetable;
_____Fruit;   _____Other Carbohydrate

AnutraSize™

SIDE DISHES

ANUTRASIZED™ GARLIC HERB PARMESAN BREAD

Makes 12 Servings

1 loaf French bread
12 tablespoons ANUTRA®
1/2 cup Anutra® Butter
1/2 cup Anutra® Garlic Herb Parmesan

Cut bread in half lengthwise. Combine Anutra® Garlic Herb Parmesan, Anutra® and Anutra® Butter. Spread over cut surfaces of bread. Place bread cut side up on a baking sheet. Broil 5 minutes or until browned/melted. This is an excellent accompaniment to any entrée.

Nutrition per serving: 172 Calories; 5.6g Fat (29% calories from fat); 7g Protein; 23.5g Carbohydrate; 0mg Cholesterol; 390mg Sodium. Exchanges: 1-1/2 Grain (Starch); 1/2 Lean Protein; 1/2 Fat.

BROWN RICE AND ANUTRA® CHEDDAR
WITH PINE NUTS

Makes 8 Servings

1-1/2 cups long-grain brown rice
4 cups water
1 onion — chopped
1 tablespoon corn oil
1 tablespoon ground cumin
black pepper — to taste
1 cup Anutra® Cheddar Shreds
1/2 cup ANUTRA®
1 tablespoon fresh parsley — minced
1/4 cup pine nuts

Soak brown rice in water at least 2 hours or overnight. Heat oil in a heavy skillet with tight-fitting lid. Add chopped onion and sauté until golden brown and limp. Add rice, Anutra® and soaking water along with cumin and pepper. Bring to a boil, reduce heat, and cover. Cook at a simmer for about 20 minutes. Rice should be tender and water should be absorbed. When rice is done, fold in Anutra® Shreds add chopped parsley and pine nuts.

Nutrition per serving: 236 Calories; 9g Fat (34% calories from fat); 8.3g Protein; 32.5g Carbohydrate; 0mg Cholesterol; 202mg Sodium. Exchanges: 2 Grain (Starch); 1/2 Lean Protein; 1/2 Vegetable; 1 Fat.

CHEESY ANUTRA® PEPPER JACK CORN BREAD

Makes 12 Servings

1/2 cup whole wheat flour
3/4 cup ANUTRA®
2 teaspoons baking powder
1 teaspoon baking soda
1/4 teaspoon salt
1 1/2 cups yellow cornmeal
1/2 cup brown sugar, packed
1/4 cup 99% fat-free egg substitute or egg whites
1 cup water
1 teaspoon canola oil
1 cup Anutra® Sour Cream
1 cup Anutra® Shreds - Pepper Jack and Cheddar Blend

Preheat oven to 350 degrees. Combine first 7 dry ingredients in a medium sized bowl. In a separate bowl, combine egg whites, canola oil, and Anutra® Sour Cream. Add the wet mixture to the dry mixture, then add the Anutra® Shreds. Mix with a wooden spoon or spatula until combined. Spread into a lightly vegetable sprayed 8 inch pan, square or round. Bake for 30-35 minutes or until center springs back.

Nutrition per serving: 194 Calories; 5.8g Fat (27% calories from fat); 29.9g Protein; 30.9g Carbohydrate; 0mg Cholesterol; 385mg Sodium. Exchanges: 1 Grain (Starch); 1/2 Lean Protein; 1/2 Fat; 1/2 Other Carbohydrates.

CONCETTA'S BAKED EGGPLANT PARMIGIANA ANUTRASIZED™

Makes 8 Servings

1 large eggplant — peeled and sliced round, cut 1/4-inch thick
6 tablespoons virgin olive oil
1 cup low sodium bread crumbs, seasoned
1/2 cup ANUTRA®
12 Anutra® Mozzarella Slices
1 cup Anutra® Shreds - Parmesan, Mozzarella & Romano Blend
1/4 cup Anutra® Parmesan Cheese
2-1/2 cups tomato sauce

Toss eggplant slices in olive oil. Coat eggplant with seasoned bread crumbs. Place slices on non-stick cookie sheet and bake at 350 degrees for 10 minutes on each side. Cover the bottom of a 6" x 10" pan with 3/4 cup of tomato sauce; add one layer of eggplant slices;sprinkle Anutra®; top with 4 slices of Anutra® Mozzarella, 1 tablespoon Anutra® Parmesan, 1/3 of the Anutra® Shreds; continue adding one layer of eggplant slices, Anutra®, Anutra® Slices, Anutra® Parmesan, Anutra® Shreds, and tomato sauce until eggplant slices are finished. Top last eggplant layer with Anutra® Slices, remaining Anutra® Parmesan, Anutra® Shreds and tomato sauce. Bake at 350 degrees for one half hour.

This is a great tasting eggplant parmigiana without all the typical fat associated with this dish.

Nutrition per serving: 311 Calories; 18.1g Fat (52% calories from fat); 14.7g Protein; 23.8g Carbohydrate; 0mg Cholesterol; 928mg Sodium. Exchanges: 1/2 Grain (Starch); 1-1/2 Lean Protein; 1-1/2 Vegetable; 2 Fat.

CONCETTA'S ANUTRA® SHREDS
WITH ROASTED PEPPERS AND SPINACH

Makes 8 Servings

10 ounces frozen spinach
1 tablespoon virgin olive oil
6 garlic cloves — peeled
12 ounces roasted red peppers in jar, drained — sliced 1/2-inch thick
1/2 cup ANUTRA®
1/2 cup Anutra® Shreds - Parmesan, Mozzarella & Romano Blend

Defrost spinach in microwave. Add olive oil to frying pan and heat to medium-high temperature. Lightly sauté the garlic; add spinach and sliced roasted peppers. Mix until heated. Take off heat and fold in Anutra® Shreds or place on top as garnish. Sprinkle with Anutra® Serve.

Nutrition per serving: 80 Calories; 4.7g Fat (53% calories from fat); 4.1g Protein; 7.4g Carbohydrate; 0mg Cholesterol; 125mg Sodium. Exchanges: 1/2 Lean Protein; 1 Vegetable; 1/2 Fat.

JERK SPICE BLACK BEAN YUKON GOLD ANUTRA® MASHED POTATOES

Makes 10 Servings

4 pounds Yukon gold potatoes — diced
3/4 cup Anutra® Butter
2/3 cup ANUTRA®
1/2 cup Anutra® Cheddar Shreds
1-1/4 cups black beans, cooked
2 teaspoons dried jerk spice
1/4 cup Anutra® Milk
pinch salt and pepper

Heat enough water (approx 1-1/2 quarts) to boil potatoes. Add diced potatoes to boiling water, cover and cook for 10-12 minutes until tender. Using a colander, drain water from potatoes. Place hot potatoes in mixing bowl, add remaining ingredients. Mash by hand or with a mixer. Serve.

Nutrition per serving: 253 Calories; 6.4g Fat (23% calories from fat); 9.2g Protein; 38.5g Carbohydrate; 0mg Cholesterol; 238mg Sodium. Exchanges: 1/2 Grain (Starch); 1/2 Fat.

POTATOES AU ANUTRA® GRATIN

Makes 12 Servings

1/4 cup low sodium vegetable broth
2 cups Anutra® Cheddar Shreds
3/4 cup Anutra® Sour Cream
1/4 cup Anutra® Butter
3/4 cup ANUTRA®
1-1/3 cup water
1/2 teaspoon garlic powder
1 teaspoon dried oregano
1/2 teaspoon dried thyme
pinch salt and pepper
1-1/4 pounds potatoes, sliced
bread crumbs
vegetable cooking spray

Preheat oven to 350 degrees. Combine all ingredients except sliced potatoes. Mix until well blended. Fold in sliced potatoes. Add mixture to lightly coated 2 quart baking dish. Top with bread crumbs and lightly add vegetable spray to top. Bake covered for 30 minutes and uncovered for 10-15 minutes until top has browned.

Nutrition per serving: 118 Calories; 4.5g Fat (34% calories from fat); 6.3g Protein; 13.4g Carbohydrate; 0mg Cholesterol; 361mg Sodium. Exchanges: 1/2 Grain (Starch); 1 Lean Protein; 1/2 Fat.

ROASTED GARLIC YUKON GOLD MASHED POTATOES ANUTRASIZED™

Makes 6 Servings

3 cups Yukon gold potato — diced
1/3 cup Anutra® Butter
6 tablespoons ANUTRA®
2/3 cups water
4 garlic cloves
1/4 cup Anutra® Milk
pinch salt and pepper
vegetable cooking spray

Heat oven to 350 degrees. Place foil on small sheet pan, place garlic cloves in the middle and lightly spray with cooking oil. Cover pan with foil and bake for 30-35 minutes until garlic is soft. Heat enough water (approx 1-1/2 quarts) to boil potatoes. Add diced potatoes to boiling water, cover and cook for 10-12 minutes until tender. Using a knife, chop and mash roasted garlic. Set aside. Using a colander, drain water from potatoes. Place hot potatoes in mixing bowl, add roasted garlic and remaining ingredients. Mash by hand or with a mixer. Serve.

Nutrition per serving: 1158 Calories; 4.8g Fat (27% calories from fat); 4.8g Protein; 23.4g Carbohydrate; 0mg Cholesterol; 120mg Sodium. Exchanges: 1/2 Grain (Starch); 1/2 Fat.

ROASTED SHALLOT ANUTRA®
MASHED POTATOES

Makes 5 Servings

2 large shallots
3 cups Yukon gold potatoes — diced
1/3 cup Anutra® Butter
1/4 cup Anutra® Milk
5 tablespoons ANUTRA®
1/2 cup water
1/2 teaspoon salt
1/4 teaspoon pepper
vegetable cooking spray

Heat oven to 350 degrees. Place foil on small sheet pan, place shallots in the middle and lightly spray with cooking spray. Cover pan with foil and bake for 30-35 minutes until garlic is soft. Heat enough water to boil potatoes. Add diced potatoes to boiling water, cover and cook for 10-12 minutes until tender. Using a small food processor, puree the roasted shallots. Set aside. Using a colander, drain water from potatoes. Place hot potatoes in mixing bowl, add roasted shallots and remaining ingredients. Mash by hand or with a mixer. Serve.

Nutrition per serving: 188 Calories; 5.3g Fat (25% calories from fat); 5.7g Protein; 28.6g Carbohydrate; 0mg Cholesterol; 359mg Sodium. Exchanges: 1/2 Grain (Starch); 1/2 Vegetable; 1/2 Fat.

VEGETABLE AND ANUTRA® PEPPER JACK RICE MEDLEY

Makes 6 Servings

1/2 cup yellow onions — minced
1/2 cup celery — finely chopped
1 garlic clove — minced
2 tablespoons olive oil
2-3/4 cups vegetable broth
2/3 cup water
1 cup long-grain brown rice
1/3 cup ANUTRA®
1/4 teaspoon salt — optional
1/4 teaspoon fresh-ground black pepper
1/2 cup carrots — peeled, diced
1/4 cup green peppers — diced
1 cup Anutra® Shreds - Pepper Jack and Cheddar Blend

Sauté onion, celery, and garlic in the olive oil. Use a heavy pan with a tight fitting lid. Add the diluted broth, brown rice, salt and pepper. Cover tightly and cook over low heat for 35-40 minutes. Stir in carrots and green peppers; cook 10-15 minutes longer. Fold in Anutra® Shreds. Serve.

Nutrition per serving: 309 Calories; 11.3g Fat (33% calories from fat); 10.6g Protein; 42.3g Carbohydrate; 0mg Cholesterol; 1121mg Sodium. Exchanges: 2-1/2 Grain (Starch); 1/2 Lean Protein; 1/2 Vegetable; 1-1/2 Fat.

ANUTRA® BLUE CHEESE POLENTA

Makes 6 Servings

2-1/2 cups low sodium vegetable broth
1 cup cornmeal
1/3 cup ANUTRA®
2/3 cup water
3 tablespoons Anutra® Butter
1/2 cup Anutra® Blue Cheese Crumbles
1 tablespoon Anutra® Parmesan Cheese

In a large saucepan over medium-high heat, bring stock to a boil. Reduce heat to medium. Add cornmeal by the tablespoon, stirring constantly to prevent lumps from forming. Continue stirring as mixture cooks (about 20 minutes). Polenta will pull away from sides of pan. Stir in Anutra® Butter, Anutra® and water. Fold in Blue Cheese Crumbles. Top with Anutra® Parmesan. Serve immediately.

Polenta can be prepared at the last minute or hours ahead. Top it with your favorite tomato sauce and sprinkle with basil.

Nutrition per serving: 196 Calories; 6g Fat (28% calories from fat); 12.6g Protein; 23.1g Carbohydrate; 0mg Cholesterol; 454mg Sodium. Exchanges: 1-1/2 Grain (Starch); 1-1/2 Lean Protein; 1/2 Fat.

ANUTRA® CHEDDAR AND HERBED POTATO SOUFFLE

Makes 10 Servings

1/4 cup low sodium vegetable broth
1/2 cup 99% fat-free egg substitute or egg whites
2/3 cup ANUTRA®
1-1/3 cups water
2 cups Anutra® Cheddar Shreds
3/4 cup Anutra® Sour Cream
1/4 cup Anutra® Butter
1/2 teaspoon garlic powder
1 teaspoon dried oregano
1/2 teaspoon dried thyme
pinch salt and pepper
1-1/4 pounds potatoes, shredded

Preheat oven to 350 degrees. Combine all ingredients except shredded potatoes. Mix until well blended. Fold in shredded potatoes. Add 1/2 cup of mixture to lightly coated non-stick cupcake baking pan. Bake for 30-35 minutes.

Nutrition per serving: 122 Calories; 7.4g Fat (55% calories from fat); 8.1g Protein; 6.7g Carbohydrate; 0mg Cholesterol; 414mg Sodium. Exchanges: 1-1/2 Lean Protein; 1/2 Fat.

ANUTRA® CHEDDAR STUFFED POTATOES

Makes 6 Servings

6 medium baking potatoes
1/3 cup ANUTRA®
2/3 cup water
1 cup Anutra® Cheddar Shreds
1-1/2 cups Anutra® Sour Cream
1/3 cup finely chopped green onions
1/4 teaspoon salt
paprika

Bake potatoes at 400 degrees for one hour or until done; let cool slightly. Cut a 1/4-inch-thick slice from the top of each baked potato; carefully scoop pulp into a bowl, leaving shells intact. Add Anutra® Cheddar Shreds, Anutra®, water and Anutra® Sour Cream to pulp and mash together; stir in green onions and salt.

Stuff shells with potato mixture and sprinkle with paprika. Place on a baking sheet and bake at 450 degrees for 15 minutes or until thoroughly heated.

Nutrition per serving: 267 Calories; 10.2g Fat (34% calories from fat); 10.2g Protein; 36.7g Carbohydrate; 0mg Cholesterol; 459mg Sodium. Exchanges: 1-1/2 Grain (Starch; 1-1/2 Lean Protein; 1 Fat.

ANUTRA® TWICE BAKED POTATO

Makes 4 Servings

2 potatoes — whole
2 cups potato — diced
1/3 cup Anutra® Butter
1/4 cup Anutra® Cheddar Shreds
1/4 cup ANUTRA®
1/2 cup water
1 shallot — chopped fine
1/2 tablespoon Anutra® Garlic Herb Parmesan

Heat oven to 350 degrees. Wash whole potatoes and place on baking sheet. Bake potatoes for 35-40 minutes at 350 degrees. Heat 2 quarts of water to boil in medium stockpot. Add diced potatoes to boiling water, cover and cook for 10-12 minutes. Take baked potatoes out of oven and let cool for 10 minutes. Turn oven up to 425 degrees. Using a knife, cut baked potatoes in half lengthwise. Using spoon, scoop inside of potato into mixing bowl, leaving potato skin intact. Using a colander, drain water from diced potatoes. Add the remaining ingredients to the mixing bowl, mix at low speed until well blended. Using a spatula, fill the potato skins with the potato mixture. Place filled potato on sheet pan. Place back in oven; bake until top becomes golden brown (10-15 minutes). Serve.

Nutrition per serving: 339 Calories; 7.2g Fat (19% calories from fat); 10.6g Protein; 60.1g Carbohydrate; 0mg Cholesterol; 291mg Sodium. Exchanges: 4 Grain (Starch); 1/2 Lean Protein; 1/2 Fat.

WHOLE WHEAT ANUTRA® BISCUITS

Makes 12 Servings

1 cup all-purpose flour
1 cup whole wheat flour
3/4 cup ANUTRA®
2 teaspoons baking powder
1/2 teaspoon baking soda
1/2 teaspoon salt
1/4 cup 99% fat-free egg substitute or egg whites
1 teaspoon canola oil
1/2 cup Anutra® Sour Cream
1/3 cup Anutra® Butter — melted
1 cup water
1/2 cup Anutra® Cheddar Shreds

Preheat oven to 400 degrees. Combine first six dry ingredients in a bowl. Combine eggs, canola oil, Anutra® Sour Cream, and melted Anutra® Butter in another bowl. Add the wet mixture to the dry, blend, add water and blend in the Anutra® Cheddar Shreds until minimally combined. Take dough out of bowl and place on floured surface; knead dough until smooth. Re-flour work surface and pat dough down to about 1/2 inch thick. Cut as you please with knife or cookie cutter. Bake on lightly sprayed cooking pan for 10-12 minutes. Serve immediately.

Nutrition per serving: 146 Calories; 5.5g Fat (34% calories from fat); 5.6g Protein; 19.7g Carbohydrate; 0mg Cholesterol; 345mg Sodium. Exchanges: 1 Grain (Starch); 1/2 Lean Protein; 1/2 Fat.

MY FAVORITE SIDE DISH- ANUTRASIZED™:

Makes _____**Servings**

Ingredients:

_____   _____
_____   _____
_____   _____
_____   _____
_____   _____
_____   _____
_____   _____

Instructions:

_____
_____
_____
_____
_____
_____
_____
_____
_____
_____
_____
_____
_____
_____
_____
_____

Nutrition per serving:
_____Calories; _____g Fat (_____% Fat Cal); _____g Protein;
_____g Carbohydrate; _____mg Cholesterol; _____mg Sodium.
Exchanges:
_____Grain (Starch); _____Lean Protein; _____Vegetable;
_____Fruit; _____Other Carbohydrate

MY 2ᴺᴰ FAVORITE SIDE DISH - ANUTRASIZED™:

Makes _____ Servings

Ingredients:

_____   _____
_____   _____
_____   _____
_____   _____
_____   _____
_____   _____
_____   _____

Instructions:

_____
_____
_____
_____
_____
_____
_____
_____
_____
_____
_____
_____
_____
_____

Nutrition per serving:
_____Calories;   _____g Fat (_____% Fat Cal);   _____g Protein;
_____g Carbohydrate;   _____mg Cholesterol;   _____mg Sodium.
Exchanges:
_____Grain (Starch);   _____Lean Protein;   _____Vegetable;
_____Fruit;   _____Other Carbohydrate

AnutraSize™

PIZZA

MAMA LISA'S ANUTRASIZED™ CALZONE

Makes 4 Servings

1 pound frozen pizza dough
2 cups Anutra® Mozzarella Shreds
4 tablespoons ANUTRA®
vegetable cooking spray

Thaw frozen dough. Divide into equal portions. Roll into rounds
1/2 inch thick. Place Anutra® Shreds and Anutra® on half of
round. Fold over and seal and let rise for 45 minutes. Spray lightly
with vegetable oil and bake at 375 degrees for 30 minutes.

For a spicier calzone, use Anutra® Shreds - Pepper Jack and
Cheddar Blend or add crushed black pepper to the Anutra® Shreds
of your choice.

Nutrition per serving: 396 Calories; 10.8g Fat (25% calories from fat); 19.9g
Protein; 53.9g Carbohydrate; 0mg Cholesterol; 783mg Sodium. Exchanges: 3
Grain (Starch); 2 Lean Protein; 1/2 Fat.

MEDITERRANEAN ANUTRA® PITA PIES

Makes 4 Servings

1 cup garbanzo beans, canned — drained
4 tablespoons ANUTRA®
1/2 cup water
2 tablespoons Anutra® Milk
2 tablespoons lemon juice
2 garlic cloves — minced
4 pita bread pockets
1 teaspoon olive oil
5 ounces frozen spinach
1 cup plum tomatoes, diced
1/2 cup red onions — diced
1/2 cup Anutra® Shreds - Parmesan, Mozzarella & Romano Blend
2 tablespoons black pitted olives — sliced

Preheat oven to 450 degrees. Place 4 pita pockets on a baking sheet and lightly brush each pocket with olive oil, bake for 5 minutes and set aside. In a large bowl, add the garbanzo beans, Anutra® Milk, Anutra®, lemon juice, water and garlic. With an electric mixer, blend until texture is smooth. Top each pita pocket with the garbanzo bean mixture. Place spinach on top of bean mixture. Sprinkle each pita with diced red onions, plum tomatoes and black olives. Top with the Anutra® Shreds. Bake in oven for approx 5-7 minutes or until the shreds soften.

Nutrition per serving: 341 Calories; 6.9g Fat (18% calories from fat); 14.5g Protein; 57.1g Carbohydrate; 0mg Cholesterol; 768mg Sodium. Exchanges: 3 Grain (Starch); 1/2 Lean Protein; 1 Vegetable; 1/2 Fat.

ROASTED VEGETABLE ANUTRA® FETA CALZONES

Makes 8 Servings

3 cups eggplant — diced, peeled
2 cups onion — chopped
1-1/2 cups mushrooms — diced
1-1/2 cups zucchini — diced
1 cup red bell peppers — diced
1/2 teaspoon pepper
1 tablespoon olive oil
1 cup Anutra® Feta Cheese Crumbles
1/2 cup Anutra® Mozzarella Shreds
1/2 cup ANUTRA®
1/2 cup water
1/2 cup chopped fresh basil
1 pound frozen white bread dough — thawed
vegetable cooking spray
1 egg white
1 tablespoon water

Combine eggplant and next 7 ingredients in a large roasting pan; stir well, and spread evenly. Bake at 425 degrees for 45 minutes, stirring every 15 minutes. Spoon vegetables into a bowl; stir in Anutra® Cheeses, Anutra®, water and basil. Divide dough into 8 equal portions. Working with 1 portion at a time (cover remaining dough to keep from drying out), roll each portion into a 7-inch circle on a lightly floured surface. Spoon 1/2 cup vegetable mixture onto half of each circle; moisten edges of dough with water. Fold dough over filling; press edges together with a fork to seal. Place calzones on a baking sheet coated with cooking spray. Combine the eggs and 1 tablespoon water; brush over calzones. Bake at 375 degrees for 20 minutes or until golden. Let cool on a wire rack. Serve warm or at room temperature.

Nutrition per serving: 271 Calories; 9.1g Fat (30% calories from fat); 15.4g Protein; 37.3g Carbohydrate; 0mg Cholesterol; 755mg Sodium. Exchanges: 1-1/2 Grain (Starch); 1-1/2 Lean Protein; 1-1/2 Vegetable; 1/2 Fat.

SPINACH AND ANUTRA® ASIAGO FRENCH BREAD PIZZA

Makes 4 Servings

2 cups torn spinach
4 tablespoons ANUTRA®
6 tablespoons water
vegetable cooking spray
1/8 teaspoon pepper
1 French bread loaf — (7-inch long)
1/4 cup tomato paste
1/4 teaspoon dried Italian seasoning
1/2 small garlic clove — minced
2 tablespoons Anutra® Asiago Cheese Crumbles

Place spinach in a large non-stick skillet coated with cooking spray; cover and cook over low heat 7 minutes or until spinach wilts, stirring occasionally. Toss with pepper and set aside. Slice roll in half lengthwise; place cut sides up on a baking sheet. Broil 2 minutes or until golden. Combine tomato paste, Italian seasoning, Anutra®, water and garlic; stir well and spread over the cut sides of bread. Top with spinach mixture and Anutra® Asiago Cheese Crumbles. Broil 2 minutes or until cheese softens.

For variety, try Anutra® Blue Cheese or Feta Crumbles in place of the Asiago flavor.

Nutrition per serving: 136 Calories; 4.1g Fat (27% calories from fat); 7.1g Protein; 20.6g Carbohydrate; 0mg Cholesterol; 516mg Sodium. Exchanges: 1/2 Grain (Starch); 1/2 Lean Protein; 1-1/2 Vegetable.

ANUTRA® BLUE CHEESE AND ONION FOCACCIA PIZZA

Makes 8 Servings

1 package dry yeast
1-1/2 cup warm water
1/4 teaspoon sugar
2 cups all-purpose flour
1/2 cup ANUTRA®
1/2 teaspoon salt
vegetable cooking spray
1 teaspoon vegetable oil
2 cups thinly sliced onion,

separated into rings
2 teaspoons chopped fresh thyme
or 1 teaspoon dried whole thyme
1/8 teaspoon salt
1/8 teaspoon pepper
1/2 cup Anutra® Cream Cheese
1 cup Anutra® Blue Cheese
Crumbles

In a small bowl, dissolve yeast in 1/4 cup warm water. Add sugar and let stand 5 minutes. In food processor, add flour and 1/2 teaspoon salt; pulse 2 times or until blended. With processor running, slowly add yeast mixture, Anutra® and remaining warm water through food chute; process until dough leaves sides of bowl and forms a ball. Process 30 additional seconds. Place dough in a large bowl coated with cooking spray, turning to coat top. Cover and let rise in a warm place (85 degrees), free from drafts, for approx 45 minutes or until doubled in size. Punch dough down, and pat into a 12-inch circle on a large baking sheet coated with cooking spray. Lightly coat dough with cooking spray. Cover dough with heavy-duty plastic wrap and let rise in a warm place (85 degrees) free from drafts, for 25 minutes or until puffy.

While dough rises, coat a large non-stick skillet with cooking spray; add oil, and place over medium-high heat until hot. Add onion; sauté 8 minutes or until onion is deep golden. Stir in thyme, salt, and pepper. Remove from heat; set aside.

Using the handle of a wooden spoon or your fingertips, make indentations in top of dough. Gently spread Anutra® Cream Cheese over dough, leaving a 1/2 inch border. Arrange onion mixture evenly over Anutra® Cream Cheese and sprinkle with Anutra® Blue Cheese Crumbles. Bake at 375 degrees for 15- 20 minutes or until crust sounds hollow when tapped. Cut focaccia into wedges and serve warm.

To save time, you can also use a store-bought focaccia crust. Just add topping and bake. If made ahead of time, wrap uncut bread in aluminum foil and reheat at 350 degrees for 15 minutes.

Nutrition per serving: 252 Calories; 7.5g Fat (27% calories from fat); 13.8g Protein; 33.2g Carbohydrate; 0mg Cholesterol; 670mg Sodium. Exchanges: 1-1/2 Grain (Starch); 1-1/2 Lean Protein; 1/2 Vegetable; 1/2 Fat.

ANUTRA® EGGPLANT AND TOMATO PIZZA

Makes 8 Servings

1 pizza crust
1 teaspoon olive oil
1 teaspoon chopped garlic
2 cups eggplant — 1/2-inch diced
1 tomato, whole — sliced 1/4-inch thick
1/2 cup ANUTRA®
1 tablespoon balsamic vinegar
5 basil leaves — torn
1 teaspoon oregano
3/4 cup pizza sauce — any brand
1 teaspoon Anutra® Parmesan Cheese
2 cups Anutra® Mozzarella Shreds

Preheat oven to 400 degrees. Place a large sauté pan over a high heat. Add olive oil and wait 30 seconds as pan heats. Add garlic and eggplant. Turn down to medium heat. Cook for 3 minutes. Add balsamic vinegar, basil and oregano. Cook until eggplant is tender, about 3 more minutes. Remove from heat and set aside until needed. Spread pizza sauce on crust to the edges and sprinkle Anutra® over it. Place 1/2 the Anutra® Mozzarella Shreds over the sauce. Spread cooked vegetables over the cheese. Sprinkle Anutra® Parmesan topping over the eggplant. Place tomato slices over pizza. Add the rest of the mozzarella shreds. Place in the oven 10-12 minutes or until the cheese is melted. Garnish with fresh basil. Cut into 8 slices.

Nutrition per serving: 209 Calories; 7.3g Fat (30% calories from fat); 6.4g Protein; 30.8g Carbohydrate; 0mg Cholesterol; 174mg Sodium. Exchanges: 2 Grain (Starch); 1 Vegetable; 1/2 Fat.

ANUTRA® PEPPER JACK AND VEGGIE® CHEDDAR MINI MEXICAN PIZZAS

Makes 6 Servings

2 cups diced unpeeled tomatoes
1/3 cup ANUTRA®
2/3 cup water
1 tablespoon minced fresh cilantro
1 tablespoon finely chopped green onions
1/2 teaspoon ground cumin
1/8 teaspoon garlic powder
1 tablespoon fresh lime juice
6 flour tortillas — (8-inch)
1-1/2 cups fat-free refried beans
3/4 cup Anutra® Shreds - Pepper Jack and Cheddar Blend

Combine first 8 ingredients in a bowl; stir well, and set aside.
Arrange tortillas on baking sheets and bake at 400 degrees for 2
minutes. Turn over tortillas and bake for an additional minute.
Spread 1/4 cup beans over each tortilla; top with 1/3 cup tomato
mixture and 2 tablespoons shreds. Bake at 400 degrees for 6 minutes or until the tortillas are crisp and cheese melts; cut into
wedges.

Nutrition per serving: 228 Calories; 6.2g Fat (24% calories from fat); 9.8g Protein;
33.9g Carbohydrate; 0mg Cholesterol; 581mg Sodium. Exchanges: 2 Grain
(Starch); 1/2 Lean Protein; 1/2 Vegetable; 1/2 Fat.

ANUTRA® PIZZA MEXICANA

Makes 8 Servings

1 pizza crust — 12-inch
1/4 cup Chipotle Puree — or 1/4 cup tomato ketchup and
Tabasco® sauce-mixed to spike ketchup — or 1/4 cup Tabasco® sauce
or diced green chilies
1/2 cup ANUTRA®
2 cups Anutra® Shreds - Pepper Jack and Cheddar Blend
1 small red onion — sliced into thin rounds
2 ripe tomatoes — cored at the top and sliced equally
1 red bell pepper or green bell pepper — cored seeded, sliced into thin
rounds
1/2 tablespoon olive oil
1 garlic clove, finely minced or pressed
fresh ground black pepper
2 teaspoons minced fresh marjoram — or oregano
2 teaspoons minced cilantro
2 tablespoons Anutra® Parmesan Cheese

Preheat oven to 400 degrees. To make the chipotle puree, take one chipotle pepper and mince or puree very finely. Thin puree to spreading consistency by mixing in olive oil, or 1/4 cup tomato ketchup and Tabasco® sauce mixed to spike ketchup, or 1/4 cup Tabasco® sauce or diced green chilies. Spread the puree evenly over the pizza crust. Sprinkle the Anutra® and Anutra® Shreds on top of the puree. Arrange the onions, tomatoes, and peppers on top of the cheese. Combine the olive oil and garlic. Drizzle it over the vegetables. Bake the pizza in the upper 1/3 of a preheated 400 degree oven for 15-20 minutes, or until the crust is brown and crisp around the edges. Remove from the oven, sprinkle with the herbs and Anutra® Parmesan. Serve.

Chipotle chili peppers are jalapeños which have been dried and smoked. They are very hot and available in cans.

Nutrition per serving: 271 Calories; 9.9g Fat (33% calories from fat); 13g Protein; 33.1g Carbohydrate; 0mg Cholesterol; 525mg Sodium. Exchanges: 2 Grain (Starch); 1 Lean Protein; 1 Vegetable; 1/2 Fat.

ANUTRA® VEGETABLE PIZZA 12-INCH

Makes 8 Servings

1 pizza crust
1 teaspoon olive oil
1 teaspoon chopped garlic
3/4 cup zucchini — 1/2-inch diced
3/4 cup yellow squash — 1/2-inch diced
3/4 cup sliced mushrooms
1/4 cup red onion — 1/2-inch diced
1/2 cup red bell peppers — 1/2-inch diced
1 tablespoon balsamic vinegar
1 teaspoon basil
1 teaspoon oregano
3/4 cup pizza sauce — any brand
1 teaspoon Anutra® Parmesan Cheese
2 cups Anutra® Mozzarella Shreds — 1- 8 ounce bag
1/2 cup ANUTRA®

Preheat oven to 450 degrees. Place a large sauté pan over high heat. Add olive oil, wait 30 seconds as pan heats. Add garlic, zucchini, yellow squash, mushrooms, onions, and peppers. Cook for 3 minutes. Add balsamic vinegar, basil and oregano. Cook until vegetables are tender, about 3 more minutes. Remove from heat and set aside until needed. Spread pizza sauce on crust to the edges and sprinkle with Anutra®. Place half of the Anutra® Shreds over the sauce. Spread cooked vegetables over the shreds. Sprinkle Anutra® Parmesan topping over the vegetables. Place the rest of the shreds on top of the vegetables. Place in oven 10-12 minutes or until the cheese is melted. Cut into 8 slices and serve.

Nutrition per serving: 210 Calories; 7.3g Fat (31% calories from fat); 7.6g Protein; 30.9g Carbohydrate; 0mg Cholesterol; 173mg Sodium. Exchanges: 2 Grain (Starch); 1 Vegetable; 1/2 Fat.

MY FAVORITE PIZZA - ANUTRASIZED™:

Makes _____ Servings

Ingredients:

_____   _____

_____   _____

_____   _____

_____   _____

_____   _____

_____   _____

_____   _____

Instructions:

_____

_____

_____

_____

_____

_____

_____

_____

_____

_____

_____

_____

_____

Nutrition per serving:
_____ Calories;   _____ g Fat (_____% Fat Cal);   _____ g Protein;
_____ g Carbohydrate;   _____ mg Cholesterol;   _____ mg Sodium.
Exchanges:
_____ Grain (Starch);   _____ Lean Protein;   _____ Vegetable;
_____ Fruit;   _____ Other Carbohydrate

MY 2ND FAVORITE PIZZA - ANUTRASIZED™:

Makes _____**Servings**

Ingredients:

_____   _____
_____   _____
_____   _____
_____   _____
_____   _____
_____   _____
_____   _____

Instructions:

_____
_____
_____
_____
_____
_____
_____
_____
_____
_____
_____
_____
_____
_____

Nutrition per serving:
_____Calories;   _____g Fat (_____% Fat Cal);   _____g Protein;
_____g Carbohydrate;   _____mg Cholesterol;   _____mg Sodium.
Exchanges:
_____Grain (Starch);   _____Lean Protein;   _____Vegetable;
_____Fruit;   _____Other Carbohydrate

AnutraSize™

SAUCES

CILANTRO ANUTRA® PESTO SAUCE

Makes 8 Servings

1 bunch fresh cilantro
1 ounce fresh parsley
1-1/2 ounces pine nuts
1/3 cup Anutra® Parmesan Cheese
1/2 cup ANUTRA®
3/4 cup water
1/2 teaspoon black pepper
1-1/2 teaspoons chopped garlic
1 tablespoon olive oil

Place cilantro and parsley into a food processor; blend until smooth. Add everything but the olive oil. Turn on food processor and slowly add oil. Blend until smooth and creamy. This recipe will produce 1 cup of sauce.

Nutrition per serving: 86 Calories; 6.8g Fat (71% calories from fat); 4.4g Protein; 3.6g Carbohydrate; 0mg Cholesterol; 86mg Sodium. Exchanges: 1/2 Lean Protein; 1 Fat.

DIJON CHEESE SAUCE ANUTRASIZED™

Makes 8 Servings

1 cup Vegan Cheddar Cheese Sauce Alternative
1/2 cup ANUTRA®
1 cup water
1 tablespoon dijon mustard
1/2 teaspoon garlic powder
1/2 dash Tabasco® sauce
1/2 dash white pepper

Place all ingredients but Anutra® in small stock pot. Heat to boil while stirring constantly. Reduce to simmer, Add Anutra® let cook for 5-7 minutes stirring as needed. Serve.

This recipe can be used on top of potatoes, vegetables, pastas, rice, and more. It may also be used as a sandwich sauce or nacho dip. As a variation, add your favorite garnish such as broccoli, stewed tomatoes, green peppers, mushrooms or beans.

Nutrition per serving: 69 Calories; 4.1g Fat (53% calories from fat); 3.1g Protein; 5.3g Carbohydrate; 0mg Cholesterol; 414mg Sodium. Exchanges: 1/2 Fat.

ANUTRASIZED™ ITALIANO CHEESE SAUCE

Makes 8 Servings

1/2 cup Vegan Cheddar Cheese Sauce Alternative
1/2 cup marinara sauce
1/2 cup ANUTRA®
1 cup water
1/4 teaspoon oregano
1/4 teaspoon thyme

Place all ingredients but Anutra® in small stock pot. Heat to boil while stirring constantly. Reduce to simmer, add Anutra® let cook for 5-7 minutes stirring as needed. Serve.

This recipe may be used on top of potatoes, vegetables, pastas, rice, and more. As a variation, add your favorite garnish like broccoli, carrots, tomatoes, black olives, green peppers, mushrooms or beans, or add fresh herbs such as basil and parsley. This recipe will produce 1 cup of sauce.

Nutrition per serving: 55 Calories; 3.1g Fat (51% calories from fat); 3.3g Protein; 5.2g Carbohydrate; 0mg Cholesterol; 226mg Sodium. Exchanges: 1/2 Vegetable; 1/2 Fat.

ANUTRASIZED™ MEXI QUESO SAUCE

Makes 8 Servings

1/2 cup Vegan Cheddar Cheese Sauce Alternative
1/2 cup ANUTRA®
1 cup water
1/2 cup salsa
1/4 teaspoon oregano
1 dash cumin

Place all ingredients but Anutra® in small stock pot. Heat to boil while stirring constantly. Reduce to simmer, add Anutra® and let cook for 5-7 minutes stirring as needed. Serve.

This recipe can be used on top of potatoes, vegetables, pastas, rice, and more. As a variation, add your favorite garnish like jalapeños, stewed tomatoes, black olives, green peppers, mushrooms, kidney and black beans.

Nutrition per serving: 51 Calories; 3.1g Fat (55% calories from fat); 3.2g Protein; 5.3g Carbohydrate; 0mg Cholesterol; 237mg Sodium. Exchanges: 1/2 Fat.

SUN-DRIED TOMATO ANUTRA® BUTTER

Makes 8 Servings

1/4 cup sun-dried tomatoes
1/3 cup Anutra® Butter
1/2 cup ANUTRA®
1 cup water
1 small shallot - chopped
1-1/2 teaspoons chopped parsley
1/4 teaspoon salt
1/4 teaspoon black pepper

Place sun-dried tomatoes in boiling water for one minute; this will make them easier to cut. Roughly chop the tomatoes and place in a food processor. Add the rest of the ingredients and blend until smooth.

Nutrition per serving: 77 Calories; 4g Fat (47% calories from fat); 3.7g Protein; 7.6g Carbohydrate; 0mg Cholesterol; 169mg Sodium. Exchanges: 1/2 Fat.

SWEET RED PEPPER ANUTRA® BUTTER

Makes 6 Servings

1/2 cup fresh red peppers - sliced
1/3 cup Anutra® Butter
1/3 cup ANUTRA®
2/3 cup water
1/2 teaspoon salt
1/4 teaspoon black pepper

Set oven on broil. Place cut peppers, skin side up, on a non-stick baking pan. Broil until skin turns black, remove from oven and peel while still warm. Place peppers in food processor and puree. Place the rest of ingredients in food processor and blend well. Place butter mixture in a container and refrigerate until service.

You may also use store bought roasted red peppers already roasted.

Nutrition per serving: 65 Calories; 4.7g Fat (65% calories from fat); 2g Protein; 4.4g Carbohydrate; 0mg Cholesterol; 285mg Sodium. Exchanges: 1/2 Grain (Starch); 1/2 Fat.

VEGAN ALFREDO SAUCE

Makes 8 Servings

1 cup Vegan White Cheese Sauce Alternative
1/2 cup ANUTRA®
1 teaspoon olive oil
2 tablespoons white wine
2 tablespoons Vegan Parmesan
1 teaspoon garlic powder
pinch black pepper

In sauce pan, add olive oil and heat to medium heat; add remaining ingredients adjusting thickness with the addition of white wine or vegetable stock.

Nutrition per serving: 79 Calories; 4.6g Fat (52% calories from fat); 3.7g Protein; 5.3g Carbohydrate; 0mg Cholesterol; 399mg Sodium. Exchanges: 1/2 Lean Protein; 1/2 Fat.

VEGAN CHEESE SAUCE FOR
MACARONI AND CHEESE

Makes 8 Servings

1 cup Vegan Cheddar Cheese Sauce Alternative
1/2 cup ANUTRA®
1 teaspoon garlic powder
1 teaspoon onion powder
1 teaspoon mustard
1/2 dash white pepper
1 drop hot sauce
1 cup water

Place all ingredients but Anutra® in small stock pot. Heat to boil while stirring constantly. Reduce to simmer, add Anutra® let cook for 5-10 minutes stirring as needed. Add cooked macaroni or pasta (2-3 cups) of choice and ladle sauce on top of macaroni or your favorite pasta. Serve.

This recipe may be used on top of potatoes, vegetables, rice, and more. As a variation, add garnish such as broccoli, stewed tomatoes, green peppers, mushrooms or beans.

Nutrition per serving: 70 Calories; 4g Fat (51% calories from fat); 3.1g Protein; 5.5g Carbohydrate; 0mg Cholesterol; 398mg Sodium. Exchanges: 1/2 Fat.

ANUTRA® CHEDDAR SAUCE

Makes 10 Servings

2 cups Anutra® Cheddar Shreds
2/3 cup ANUTRA®
3/4 cup low sodium vegetable broth
1 cup water
1/2 teaspoon garlic powder
1/2 teaspoon cornstarch
2 tablespoons low sodium vegetable broth

In a medium stock pot over medium heat, add Anutra® Shreds, 1 cup diluted vegetable broth and garlic powder stirring constantly. In a separate small bowl, combine cornstarch, Anutra® and remaining broth. Slowly add to shred sauce and continue to cook for 5 minutes at same heat. Add more broth as needed to achieve desired thickness.

Nutrition per serving: 80 Calories; 4.4g Fat (50% calories from fat); 6.8g Protein; 4g Carbohydrate; 0mg Cholesterol; 336mg Sodium. Exchanges: 1 Lean Protein.

ANUTRA® GARLIC HERB BUTTER

Makes 8 Servings

1/2 cup Anutra® Butter
1/2 cup ANUTRA®
2 teaspoons chopped garlic
1 teaspoon fresh basil — chopped
1/4 teaspoon fresh oregano — chopped
1/2 teaspoon fresh thyme — chopped
1 teaspoon fresh parsley — chopped
1/2 teaspoon chopped shallots

Place all ingredients in a food processor and blend well. Place in a container and refrigerate until needed.

This recipe may be used with any kind of pasta or vegetables.

Nutrition per serving: 68 Calories; 5g Fat (66% calories from fat); 2.1g Protein; 4.3g Carbohydrate; 0mg Cholesterol; 120mg Sodium. Exchanges: 1/2 Grain (Starch); 1/2 Fat.

ANUTRA® PESTO SAUCE

Makes 8 Servings

1/2 cup fresh basil — packed
1/2 cup fresh parsley — packed
1/2 cup ANUTRA®
3/4 cup water
1/4 cup pine nuts — toasted
3/8 cup Anutra® Parmesan Cheese
1/2 teaspoon black pepper
1 tablespoon chopped garlic
1/2 teaspoon salt
1/4 cup low sodium vegetable broth
1/4 cup olive oil

Place basil and parsley into a food processor; blend for 30 seconds. Add everything but the olive oil to the bowl. Turn on food processor; blend for 1 minute. Add olive oil and blend until smooth.

Nutrition per serving: 138 Calories; 12g Fat (78% calories from fat); 4.9g Protein; 4.9g Carbohydrate; 0mg Cholesterol; 278mg Sodium. Exchanges: 1/2 Lean Protein; 2 Fat.

ANUTRA® RAREBIT SAUCE

Makes 10 Servings

1 cup Anutra® Milk
2/3 cup ANUTRA®
1-1/3 cup water
1-3/4 cups Anutra® Cheddar Shreds
1 dash white pepper
2 drops Tabasco® sauce
1/2 teaspoon Worcestershire sauce
1 dash cayenne pepper
2 tablespoons light beer

Heat Anutra® Milk and water on medium-high heat; do not bring to a boil. Whisk in cheddar shreds until completely melted. Add white pepper, Tabasco®, Worcestershire sauce, and cayenne pepper. Mix well. Add Anutra® and mix well. Add beer and cook 3-5 minutes longer on medium heat. Serve over vegetables or a baked potato. This recipe will produce 2-1/2 cups of sauce.

Nutrition per serving: 81 Calories; 4.4g Fat (49% calories from fat); 6.1g Protein; 4.8g Carbohydrate; 0mg Cholesterol; 289mg Sodium. Exchanges: 1 Lean Protein.

ANUTRASIZED™ WHITE WINE AND BASIL CHEESE SAUCE

Makes 8 Servings

1 cup Vegan White Cheese Sauce Alternative
1/2 cup ANUTRA®
1 cup water
1/4 cup white wine
1/2 teaspoon basil
1/4 teaspoon garlic powder
1/2 dash white pepper

Place all ingredients in small stock pot. Heat to boil while stirring constantly. Reduce to simmer, let cook for 5-7 minutes stirring as needed. Serve.

This recipe may be used on top of potatoes, vegetables, pastas, rice, and more. As a variation, add 1 cup of your favorite garnish such as broccoli, stewed tomatoes, sun-dried tomatoes, green peppers, mushrooms, pine nuts or beans.

Nutrition per serving: 73 Calories; 4g Fat (49% calories from fat); 3g Protein; 5.2g Carbohydrate; 0mg Cholesterol; 390mg Sodium. Exchanges: 1/2 Fat.

AnutraSize™

DESSERTS

ANUTRASIZED™ PUMPKIN PIE

Makes 8 Servings

1 pie crust — 9-inch, uncooked
1/8 teaspoon salt
2/3 cup sugar
2 teaspoons pumpkin pie spice
3 egg whites — slightly beaten
1-2/3 cups Anutra® Milk
1-1/2 cups pumpkin — mashed
1/2 cup ANUTRA®
1 cup water

Preheat oven to 450 degrees. Sift dry ingredients together. Stir in eggs, and mix well. Add pumpkin, Anutra®, water and Anutra® Milk. Mix well. Place mix into pie shell and bake for 10 minutes. Reduce heat to 325 degrees and bake for 35-45 minutes, or until a toothpick comes out clean. Let cool on rack.

Nutrition per serving: 228 Calories; 8.7g Fat (34% calories from fat); 5.8g Protein; 33.3g Carbohydrate; 0mg Cholesterol; 227mg Sodium. Exchanges: 1 Grain (Starch); 1 Lean Protein; 1 Fruit; 1 Fat; 1 Other Carbohydrate.

ANGELO'S ANUTRA® BUTTERCREAM FROSTING

Makes 24 Servings

1/2 cup Anutra® Butter
3/4 cup Anutra® Cream Cheese
1 teaspoon vanilla extract
3/4 cup confectioners sugar

Place all ingredients in bowl. Whip until well combined.

As a variation, add 1/4 cup cocoa powder for Anutra® Chocolate Buttercream Frosting or 1 tablespoon of Grand Marnier for Anutra® Grand Marnier Chocolate Buttercream Frosting or add any of your favorite liquors, flavors or fruits.

Nutrition per serving: 41 Calories; 1.8g Fat (38% calories from fat); 1.6g Protein; 5g Carbohydrate; 0mg Cholesterol; 95mg Sodium. Exchanges: 1/2 Fat; 1/2 Other Carbohydrate.

CHOCOLATE ARBORIO ANUTRA®
RICE PUDDING

Makes 24 Servings

4 cups Anutra® Milk
1-1/2 cups ANUTRA®
4 cups water
1 cup Arborio rice
1/4 cup sugar
1/2 cup cocoa powder
1/2 tablespoon vanilla extract
1/2 teaspoon cinnamon
pinch salt

Place Anutra® Milk, water, and rice in a medium sized cooking pan. Bring to a boil over direct heat, allow to simmer add Anutra® and cook for 45 minutes. Stir periodically to prevent scorching. Add remaining ingredients. Transfer rice to casserole dish and allow to cool. Serve warm or cold.

Nutrition per serving: 205 Calories; 4g Fat (18% calories from fat); 8.2g Protein; 36.4g Carbohydrate; 0mg Cholesterol; 72mg Sodium. Exchanges: 2 Grain (Starch); 1/2 Lean Protein; 1/2 Fruit; 1/2 Other Carbohydrate.

CHOCOLATE COCOA ANUTRA® CAKE

Makes 16 Servings

CAKE:
1-1/2 cups cake flour — sifted
1 cup ANUTRA®
2 cups water
1 teaspoon baking soda
1 teaspoon salt
1 cup Anutra® Butter
1 tablespoon canola oil
1/2 cup cocoa powder
1-1/3 cups granulated sugar
3/4 cup 99% fat-free egg substitute or egg whites
1 teaspoon vanilla extract
1/2 cup Anutra® Milk

FROSTING:
3/4 cup ANGELO'S ANUTRA® BUTTERCREAM
  FROSTING (see recipe page 310)
1/4 cup cocoa powder
1 tablespoon confectioners sugar
1/2 teaspoon vanilla extract

Preheat oven to 350 degrees. In a mixing bowl, combine the sugar, oil, and Anutra® Butter. Cream together well. Add the salt and the vanilla. Add Anutra® gel (soaked Anutra® and water) and mix well. Add the egg whites slowly while beating the batter. Mix well. Blend in the Anutra® Milk. Sift together the flour, cocoa and baking soda. Blend this into the cake batter. Mix together well. Pour batter into two 8 inch cake pans or one 13" x 9" pan. Bake at 350 degrees for approx 35 minutes or until done. Remove from oven and cool on rack for 30 minutes. In a medium sized bowl, combine ingredients for frosting. Add frosting to cake. Serve.

Nutrition per serving: 227 Calories; 8.3g Fat (33% calories from fat); 6.1g Protein; 34.7g Carbohydrate; 0mg Cholesterol; 439mg Sodium. Exchanges: 1 Grain (Starch); 1 Fat; 1 Other Carbohydrate.

CINNAMON RAISIN ANUTRA® MILK RICE PUDDING

Makes 4 Servings

2 cups Anutra® Milk
4 tablespoon ANUTRA®
1/2 cup water
1/4 cup white rice
1/3 cup sugar
1/2 cup raisins
1/2 teaspoon cinnamon

Pour Anutra® Milk and water into a stove-top pot. Add sugar and heat on medium heat until sugar dissolves. Add rice and Anutra® and bring to a simmer on low heat. Stir frequently to avoid rice and Anutra® from sticking to the bottom of the pan. Keep simmering over low heat for approx 35-45 minutes. Once the rice is almost finished cooking, stir in the raisins. Continue to simmer the mixture for 10 minutes so that the rice is completely cooked and has a soft to mushy texture. Remove from heat and allow to cool for 10 minutes. Sprinkle with cinnamon. Serve warm or allow to chill for 2-3 hours and serve cold.

Nutrition per serving: 244 Calories; 3.4g Fat (13% calories from fat); 6.9g Protein; 49g Carbohydrate; 0mg Cholesterol; 68mg Sodium. Exchanges: 1 Grain (Starch); 1/2 Lean Protein; 2 Fruit; 1 Other Carbohydrate.

ANUTRASIZED™ PEANUT BUTTER PIE

Makes 10 Servings

1 graham cracker pie crust, 9-inch - or
  ANUTRA® GRAHAM CRACKER CRUST (see recipe page 324)
8 ounces Anutra® Cream Cheese
8 ounces 25% less fat creamy peanut butter
4 ounces Anutra® Butter
6 ounces sugar
1/2 ounce vanilla extract
8 ounces non-dairy whipped topping — frozen and thawed

In an electric mixing bowl, combine the Anutra® Cream Cheese, peanut butter, Anutra® Butter, sugar, and vanilla extract. Cream together well. Take defrosted non-dairy whipped topping and fold into peanut butter mixture. Spread mixture into prepared pie shell. Freeze over night. Garnish with whipped topping, nuts, and chocolate cookie crumbs as desired.

Nutrition per serving: 355 Calories; 17.8g Fat (45% calories from fat); 10.5g Protein; 38.4g Carbohydrate; 0mg Cholesterol; 395mg Sodium. Exchanges: 1 Grain (Starch); 1 Lean Protein; 1 Fruit; 3 Fat; 1 Other Carbohydrate.

ANUTRA® POUND CAKE

Makes 16 Servings

2 cups cake flour — sifted
1-1/2 teaspoons baking powder
1/2 teaspoon salt
1 cup Anutra® Butter
1 cup ANUTRA®
3/4 cup water
1-1/2 teaspoons vanilla extract
1-1/4 cups sugar
3/4 cup 99% fat-free egg substitute or egg whites
1/2 cup Anutra® Milk

Sift the flour, baking powder, Ground Anutra® and salt together; set aside. Cream butter with extract. Gradually add sugar and water creaming until fluffy. Add eggs in thirds, beating thoroughly after each addition. Beating only until smooth after each addition, alternately add dry ingredients in thirds and Anutra® Milk in halves to creamed mixture. Turn batter into a greased 9-inch cake pan. Bake at 325 degrees for about 40 minutes or until cake tests done. Cool 10 minutes in pan on wire rack; remove and cool completely. Serve with a fresh fruit topping.

Nutrition per serving: 186 Calories; 5.2g Fat (25% calories from fat); 4.3g Protein; 31.1g Carbohydrate; 0mg Cholesterol; 241mg Sodium. Exchanges: 1 Grain (Starch); 1 Fruit; 1/2 Fat; 1 Other Carbohydrate.

ANUTRA® APPLE, BLUEBERRY, RAISIN AND CINNAMON COBBLER

Makes 9 Servings

6 phyllo dough sheets
vegetable cooking spray
3 cups Anutra® Blueberry Yogurt
9 tablespoon ANUTRA®
1 cup water
4 tablespoons tapioca
1/2 cup sugar
1 quart apple slices — drained
1 cup raisins, seedless
1 cup low-fat granola
1 tablespoon brown sugar
2 tablespoons Anutra® Butter

Lightly spray 9" x 9" baking pan with vegetable cooking spray. Place phyllo sheets around pan lightly spraying cooking spray between each layer. Place in 350 degree oven for 5 minutes to slightly brown. Mix Anutra®, Anutra® Yogurt, tapioca, water and sugar in medium mixing bowl. Fold in drained apples and raisins. Place mixture in baked phyllo pan. Mix granola, brown sugar and Anutra® Butter. Sprinkle on top of cobbler and place in oven for 45-50 minutes. Let set for 15 minutes. Serve.

Nutrition per serving: 316 Calories; 4.7g Fat (13% calories from fat); 5.7g Protein; 65.3g Carbohydrate; 0mg Cholesterol; 143mg Sodium. Exchanges: 1-1/2 Grain (Starch); 1/2 Lean Protein; 2 Fruit; 1 Other Carbohydrate.

ANUTRA® APPLE, RAISIN AND STRAWBERRY YOGURT PIE

Makes 10 Servings

1 pie crust - 9-inch
20 ounces apple slices — canned, drained
2/3 cups ANUTRA®
1 cup Anutra® Strawberry Yogurt
2 tablespoons tapioca
1/2 cup sugar
1/2 cup raisins
2 teaspoons apple pie spice
1 cup low-fat granola
1 tablespoon brown sugar
2 tablespoons Anutra® Butter
1-1/3 cups water

Preheat oven to 400 degrees. In a large bowl, combine apple slices, Anutra®, Anutra® Strawberry Yogurt, tapioca, sugar, raisins apple pie spice and water. Mix well. Fill pie crust. In a small bowl, mix granola, brown sugar, and Anutra® Butter. Sprinkle on top of pie. Place in oven and bake for 35-45 minutes. Let cool on rack. Serve warm or cold.

Nutrition per serving: 344 Calories; 10.3g Fat (27% calories from fat); 4.9g Protein; 61.5g Carbohydrate; 0mg Cholesterol; 225mg Sodium. Exchanges: 1-1/2 Grain (Starch); 2 Fruit; 1-1/2 Fat; 1 Other Carbohydrate.

ANUTRA® BANANA CREAM PIE

Makes 8 Servings

1 ripe banana
2-1/2 cups Anutra® Milk
1 banana — diced
4 ounces non-dairy whipped topping
1 reduced fat graham cracker crust- or
  ANUTRA® GRAHAM CRACKER CRUST (see recipe page 324)
2 packages Jell-o sugar-free vanilla instant pudding

Puree very ripe banana in a small food processor. Prepare pudding according to package directions for pie using Anutra® Milk and banana puree. Once the pudding thickens, add diced bananas and pour into pie shell. Chill for 2 hours before finishing the pie. Top with non-dairy whipped topping and garnish.

Nutrition per serving: 265 Calories; 10.9g Fat (37% calories from fat); 5.3g Protein; 35.6g Carbohydrate; 0mg Cholesterol; 228mg Sodium. Exchanges: 1-1/2 Grain (Starch); 1/2 Lean Protein; 1/2 Fruit; 2 Fat.

ANUTRA® BERRIED
CHEESECAKE MOUSSE

Makes 12 Servings

1 cup Anutra® Cream Cheese
1/4 cup Anutra® Sour Cream
1/2 cup sugar
2 tablespoons Anutra® Milk
1 teaspoon vanilla extract
3/4 cup non-dairy whipped topping — frozen and thawed
2 cups strawberries — quartered
2 cups raspberries
2 cups blackberries
2 cups blueberries
3/4 cup ANUTRA®

Cream sugar, Anutra® Sour Cream, and Anutra® Cream Cheese together until mixed well. Add Anutra® Milk and mix well. Add vanilla extract; mix well. Set aside. Fold in non-dairy whipped topping. Fold in fresh or frozen berries. You may also place fresh or thawed berries on top. Spoon into glasses and serve. Sprinkle Anutra® over each glass at a rate of one tablespoon per cup.

Nutrition per serving: 191 Calories; 7.7g Fat (36% calories from fat); 5.3g Protein; 26.7g Carbohydrate; 0mg Cholesterol; 158mg Sodium. Exchanges: 1/2 Lean Protein; 1 Fruit; 1 Fat; 1/2 Other Carbohydrate.

ANUTRA® CARROT CAKE

Makes 9 Servings

CAKE:
1/2 cup Anutra® Butter
1 cup sugar
1/2 cup 99% fat-free egg substitute or egg whites
3/4 cup all-purpose flour
9 tablespoons ANUTRA®
1 cup water
1/2 teaspoon baking soda
1/2 teaspoon salt
1/2 teaspoon cinnamon
1/2 teaspoon vanilla extract
1/2 cup crushed pineapple — drained
1 cup shredded carrots

FROSTING:
ANGELO'S ANUTRA® BUTTERCREAM
  FROSTING (see recipe page 310)

Heat oven to 350 degrees. In mixing bowl, combine all purpose flour, Anutra®, baking soda, salt, and cinnamon. Set aside. In separate bowl, cream Anutra® Butter and sugar. Slowly add eggs. Add flour mixture and combine. Add water. Fold in pineapple and shredded carrots. Place mixture in sprayed 9" x 9" baking pan and bake for 25-30 minutes. Let cool on rack for 25-30 minutes before serving. Top with ANGELO'S ANUTRA® BUTTERCREAM FROSTING (see recipe page 310).

Nutrition per serving: 207 Calories; 4.8g Fat (21% calories from fat); 4.2g Protein; 37.7g Carbohydrate; 0mg Cholesterol; 319mg Sodium. Exchanges: 1 Grain (Starch); 1-1/2 Fruit; 1/2 Fat; 1-1/2 Other Carbohydrate.

ANUTRA® COCOA BROWNIES

Makes 24 Servings

BROWNIE:
2 cups all-purpose flour
1-1/2 cups ANUTRA®
1-1/2 cups water
2 teaspoons baking soda
1/4 teaspoon salt
1 cup Anutra® Butter
1 tablespoon canola oil
3/4 cup cocoa powder
2 cups sugar
1 cup 99% fat-free egg substitute or egg whites
2 teaspoons vanilla extract

FROSTING:
1-1/2 cups ANGELO'S ANUTRA® BUTTERCREAM FROSTING
  (see recipe page 310)
1/4 cup cocoa powder
1 teaspoon vanilla extract

Preheat oven to 350 degrees. In a mixing bowl, combine Anutra®, flour, baking soda, and salt. Set aside. In a separate bowl, cream together sugar and Anutra® Butter. Add eggs and vanilla extract. Add water and mix together well. Add cocoa powder and mix well. Add dry ingredients 1/3 at a time and mix until a smooth batter is formed. Spread into a parchment lined pan and bake at 325 degrees for approx 30 minutes or until cake springs back. In separate bowl, combine frosting ingredients. After cake has cooled, put icing on top and cut.

Nutrition per serving: 219 Calories; 7.4g Fat (30% calories from fat); 6g Protein; 34.3g Carbohydrate; 0mg Cholesterol; 337mg Sodium. Exchanges: 1 Grain (Starch); 1 Fruit; 1/2 Fat; 1-1/2 Other Carbohydrates.

ANUTRA® CRAN-CHERRY YOGURT PIE

Makes 8 Servings

1 pie crust - 9-inch
1/2 cup ANUTRA®
1 cup water
30 ounces cherries in water — canned, drained
1 cup Anutra® Peach Yogurt
2 tablespoons tapioca
1/2 cup sugar
1/2 cup Craisins®
1 cup low-fat granola
1 tablespoon brown sugar
2 tablespoons Anutra® Butter

Preheat oven to 425 degrees. Place cookie sheet in oven while pre-heating. Combine Anutra®, drained cherries, Anutra® Yogurt, tapioca, and sugar in bowl. Mix and add water until smooth. Add cherries. Pour into frozen pie crust. Mix granola and Anutra® Butter together. Sprinkle on top of pie. Place in oven on top of cookie sheet and bake for 35-45 minutes. Remove from oven and let set for 1 hour. Serve.

Nutrition per serving: 349 Calories; 10.1g Fat (26% calories from fat); 5.3g Protein; 62.4g Carbohydrate; 0mg Cholesterol; 225mg Sodium. Exchanges: 1-1/2 Grain (Starch); 1-1/2 Fruit; 1-1/2 Fat; 1 Other Carbohydrate.

ANUTRA® CREAM CHEESE CAKE

Makes 12 Servings

24 ounces Anutra® Cream Cheese — 3 containers
8 ounces Anutra® Sour Cream — 1 container
1-3/4 cups sugar
1 cup 99% fat-free egg substitute or egg whites
1 cup Anutra® Milk
1/4 cup all-purpose flour
1/4 cup cornstarch
2 teaspoons lemon juice
1 tablespoon vanilla extract
1/4 teaspoon coconut flavoring
1 ANUTRA® GRAHAM CRACKER CRUST (see recipe page 324)

Heat oven to 325 degrees. Make Anutra® Graham Cracker Crust and place on bottom of 10-inch spring pan. Set aside. In mixing bowl, combine Anutra® Cream Cheese, Anutra® Sour Cream, and sugar. Mix well. Slowly add remaining ingredients. Mix for 3 minutes until ingredients are well combined. Pour in spring pan. Place cake on roasting pan with 3 inch sides. Pour 3/4 inch water around pan and bake for 1 hour and 30 minutes. Let cool before eating.

Nutrition per serving: 411 Calories; 13g Fat (28% calories from fat); 15.9g Protein; 61.6g Carbohydrate; 0mg Cholesterol; 665mg Sodium. Exchanges: 1-1/2 Grain (Starch); 1-1/2 Lean Protein; 2 Fruit; 1-1/2 Fat; 2 Other Carbohydrates.

ANUTRA® GRAHAM CRACKER CRUST

Makes 1 crust

1-1/4 cups graham cracker crumbs
1/3 cup ANUTRA®
1/3 cup water
2 tablespoons sugar
1/2 cup Anutra® Butter
2 tablespoons egg whites

Combine all the ingredients in a medium-sized bowl until thoroughly blended. Pack mixture firmly into pie pan and press firmly on bottom. Bake in oven at 350 degree for 7 minutes. Add filling.

Nutrition per serving: 137 Calories; 6.3g Fat (41% calories from fat); 3.3g Protein; 17.2g Carbohydrate; 0mg Cholesterol; 206mg Sodium. Exchanges: 1 Grain (Starch); 1 Fat.

ANUTRA® KEY LIME PIE

Makes 8 Servings

1/2 cup Anutra® Cream Cheese
1/2 cup Anutra® Sour Cream
4 ounces lime juice
3 tablespoons cornstarch
4 egg whites
1 cup powdered sugar
1 ANUTRA® GRAHAM CRACKER CRUST (see recipe page 324)

Place Anutra® Cream Cheese, Anutra® Sour Cream, and powdered sugar in a food processor for 1 minute. Add eggs and mix for 30 seconds more. Place Anutra® Cream Cheese mixture in a sauce pan over high heat on stove, stirring constantly for 6 minutes or until hot to the touch. Mix cornstarch with lime juice and add to the pot. Continue to stir constantly for about 2-3 minutes until very thick. Pour into pie shell and refrigerate for at least 2-3 hours. Serve cold.

Nutrition per serving: 269 Calories; 10.2g Fat (34% calories from fat); 6.9g Protein; 38.2g Carbohydrate; 0mg Cholesterol; 267mg Sodium. Exchanges: 1 Grain (Starch); 1/2 Lean Protein; 1-1/2 Fat; 1 Other Carbohydrate.

ANUTRA® MILK COCOA PUDDING CAKE

Makes 9 Servings

1 cup all-purpose flour
3/4 cup sugar
2 tablespoons unsweetened cocoa
1/4 teaspoon salt
1-1/2 teaspoons baking powder
9 tablespoon ANUTRA®
3/4 cup Anutra® Butter
1 teaspoon vanilla extract
1 cup firmly packed brown sugar
1/4 cup unsweetened cocoa
1-3/4 cups Anutra® Milk
1 cup water

Combine first 6 ingredients in a mixing bowl and stir well. Add
Anutra® Butter, Anutra® Milk, water and vanilla; stir until smooth.
Spray 9 inch baking pan and spread batter on bottom of pan.
Combine brown sugar and 1/4 cup cocoa; sprinkle over batter. Pour
boiling Anutra® Milk over batter (do not stir). Bake at 350 degrees
for 40 minutes or until cake springs back when lightly touched in
center. Serve warm.

Nutrition per serving: 318 Calories; 7g Fat (20% calories from fat); 6.2g Protein;
60.6g Carbohydrate; 0mg Cholesterol; 317mg Sodium. Exchanges: 1-1/2 Grain
(Starch); 1 Fruit; 1/2 Fat; 2-1/2 Other Carbohydrates.

ANUTRA® NUTTY BROWNIES

Makes 24 Servings

2 cups all-purpose flour
1-1/2 cup ANUTRA®
2 cups water
2 teaspoons baking soda
1/4 teaspoon salt
1 cup Anutra® Butter
1 tablespoon canola oil
3/4 cup cocoa powder
2 cups sugar
1 cup 99% fat-free egg substitute or egg whites
2 teaspoons vanilla extract
1/4 cup walnuts — chopped
2 tablespoons almonds — chopped

Preheat oven to 350 degrees. In a mixing bowl, combine flour, baking soda, and salt. Set aside. In a separate bowl, cream together sugar, Anutra® Butter, Anutra®. Add eggs and vanilla extract. Add water and mix well. Add cocoa powder and mix well. Add dry ingredients 1/3 at a time and mix until a smooth batter is formed. Fold in chopped nuts. Spread into a parchment lined pan and bake at 325 degrees for approx 30 minutes or until cake springs back. Let brownies cool on rack or eat warm.

Nutrition per serving: 185 Calories; 6.2g Fat (30% calories from fat); 4.5g Protein; 30g Carbohydrate; 0mg Cholesterol; 222mg Sodium. Exchanges: 1 Grain (Starch); 1 Fruit; 1/2 Fat; 1 Other Carbohydrate.

ANUTRA® OATMEAL RAISIN COOKIES

Makes 20 Servings

1 cup Anutra® Butter
1 teaspoon canola oil
1-1/2 cups brown sugar
1/2 cup sugar
1/4 teaspoon vanilla
1/2 cup 99% fat-free egg substitute or egg whites
2 cups water
1/2 teaspoon cinnamon
1/2 teaspoon baking soda
1 pinch salt
2 cups flour
1 cup low-fat granola
1/2 cup raisins
1 cup Quaker® oatmeal
1-1/3 cups ANUTRA®
vegetable cooking spray

Preheat oven to 350 degrees. In large mixing bowl, cream sugars, Anutra® Butter, water and oil. Add eggs and vanilla and mix well. In a medium sized mixing bowl, combine all the dry ingredients. Add the dry ingredients to the wet. Scoop out 1/4 cup servings and place on sprayed baking sheet. Bake for approx 20-25 minutes depending on thickness of cookie.

Nutrition per serving: 236 Calories; 5.3g Fat (20% calories from fat); 4.7g Protein; 43.8g Carbohydrate; 0mg Cholesterol; 203mg Sodium. Exchanges: 1 Grain (Starch); 1/2 Fruit; 1/2 Fat; 1-1/2 Other Carbohydrates.

ANUTRA® YOGURT BLUEBERRY PIE

Makes 8 Servings

1 pie crust - 9-inch
1/2 cup ANUTRA®
20 ounces blueberries in light syrup — drained
1 cup Anutra® Blueberry Yogurt
5 tablespoons tapioca
1/4 cup sugar
1 cup low-fat granola
2 tablespoons Anutra® Butter
1 cup water

Preheat oven to 425 degrees. Place cookie sheet in oven while pre-heating. Combine drained blueberries, Anutra®, Anutra® Yogurt, tapioca, sugar, and water in bowl. Mix until smooth. Add blueberries. Pour into frozen pie crust. Mix granola and Anutra® Butter together. Sprinkle on top of pie. Place in oven and bake for 35-45 minutes. Remove from oven and let set for 1 hour. Serve.

Make your favorite pie by substituting any fruit and a Anutra® Yogurt flavor of your choice.

Nutrition per serving: 317 Calories; 10g Fat (28% calories from fat); 4.5g Protein; 52.9g Carbohydrate; 0mg Cholesterol; 226mg Sodium. Exchanges: 2 Grain (Starch); 1/2 Fruit; 1-1/2 Fat; 1/2 Other Carbohydrate.

MY FAVORITE DESSERT - ANUTRASIZED™:

Makes _____ Servings

Ingredients:

_____   _____

_____   _____

_____   _____

_____   _____

_____   _____

_____   _____

_____   _____

Instructions:

_____

_____

_____

_____

_____

_____

_____

_____

_____

_____

_____

_____

_____

_____

_____

Nutrition per serving:
_____Calories;   _____g Fat (_____% Fat Cal);   _____g Protein;
_____g Carbohydrate;   _____mg Cholesterol;   _____mg Sodium.
Exchanges:
_____Grain (Starch);   _____Lean Protein;   _____Vegetable;
_____Fruit;   _____Other Carbohydrate

INDEX

INDEX (continued)

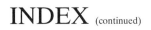

INDEX (continued)

ABOUT THE AUTHOR

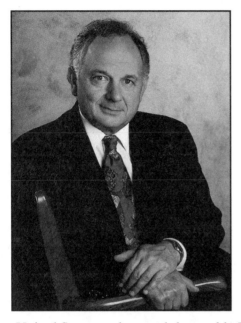

Angelo S. Morini, Founder and Chairman of Anutra® Farms, Chairman of ValuHealth, Chairman of LifeMax and Founder and Chairman Emeritus of Galaxy Nutritional Foods a publicly traded company where he invented a healthier and better way of making dairy products from a vegetable base that have been sold in over 30 countries and is the number one brand world-wide.

Mr. Morini initiated the cholesterol, low-fat, trans-fat and lactose free movement in the United States and around the world. He produced COOKING WITH THE STARS on television and, through his guest appearances on various programs and on the lecture circuit, is highly regarded as a leading crusader for healthier eating to reduce the risk of heart disease, cancer, diabetes, and many other serious maladies. His new book on **ANUTRA®**, dramatically improves your diet, reduces your intake of harmful fats and excessive calories, but not the flavor of your favorite foods, and, in the process, eliminates over 150,000 calories annually which may result in as much as a 35 pound weight loss or more. He is also active in the sociological aspects of diet and its relation to saving the precious resources of our planet and alleviating world hunger. Mr. Morini has served on President George W. Bush's Business Advisory Council.

NATURE'S BEST KEPT SECRET "ANUTRA®" WORLD'S HEALTHIEST WHOLE FOOD is his third book and it follows the successful Veggiesizing and EAT TO YOUR HEART'S CONTENT books. Mr. Morini resides with his family in Windermere, Florida.

AnutraSizing™
Recipe
Photos

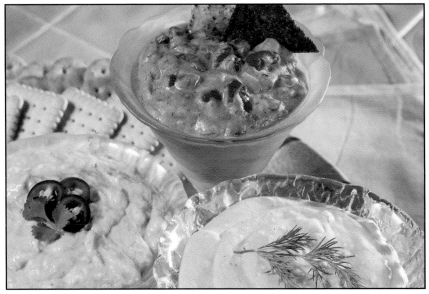

Anutra® Chili Dip - page 165; Anutra® Vegetable Guacamole - page 170; Anutra® Roasted Red Pepper Dip - page 168

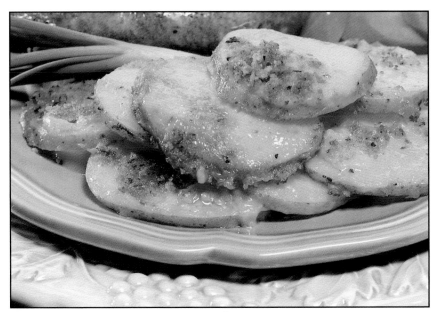

Potatoes Au Anutra® Gratin - page 268

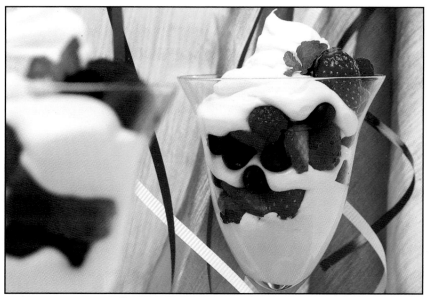

Anutra® Berried Cheesecake Mousse - page 316

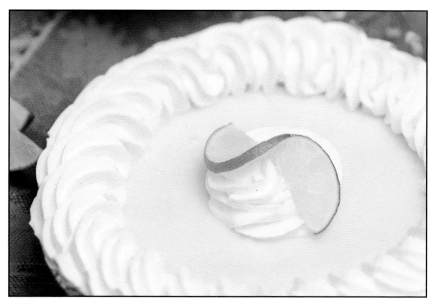

Anutra® Key Lime Pie - page 322

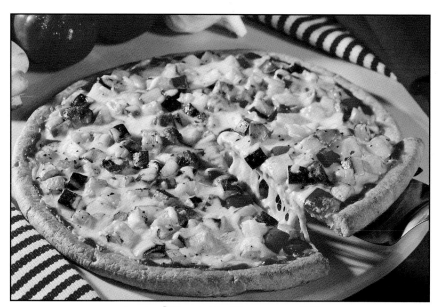

Anutra® Vegetable Pizza - page 288

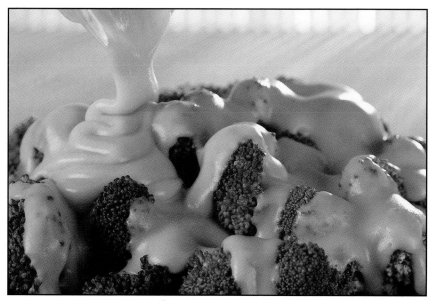

Anutra® Cheddar Sauce - page 300

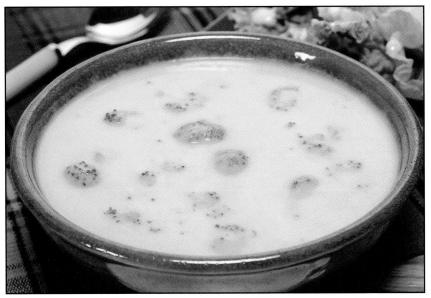

Anutra® Pepper Jack and Broccoli Soup - page 211

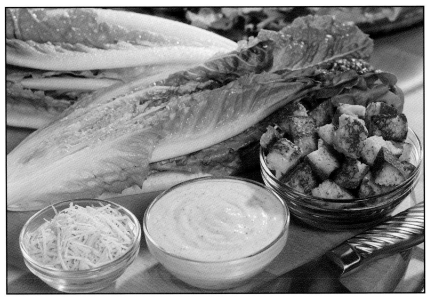

"Anutrasized™" Caesar Salad - page 174

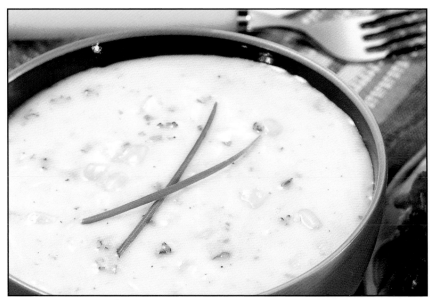

Anutra® Pepper Jack and Corn Chowder - page 210

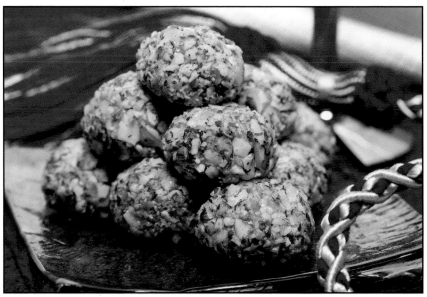

Port and Anutra® Cheddar Balls - page 157

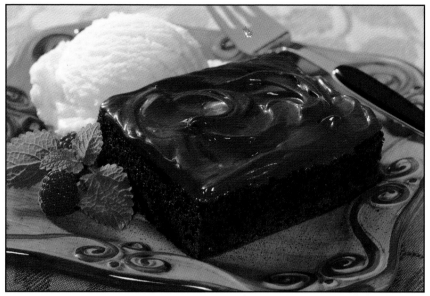

Anutra® Cocoa Brownies - page 318

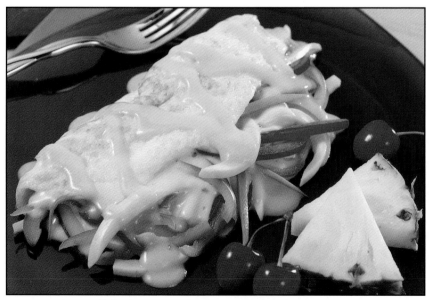

Anutra® Spring Vegetable Egg White Omelet - page 136

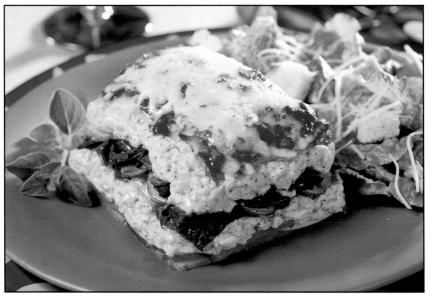

Anutra® Feta and Vegetable Lasagna- page 243

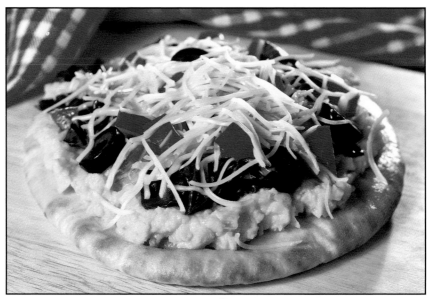

Mediterranean Anutra® Pita Pies - page 281

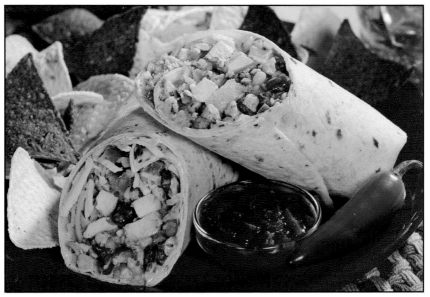

Anutra® Southwestern Vegetable Wraps - page 191

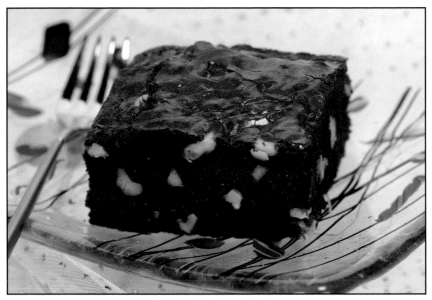

Anutra® Nutty Brownies - page 324

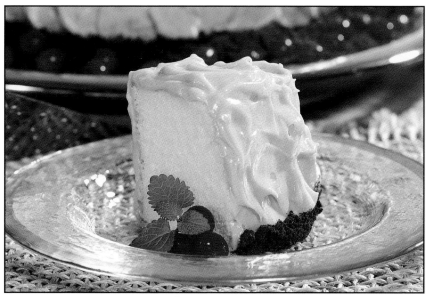

Angelo's Anutra® Buttercream Icing - page 307

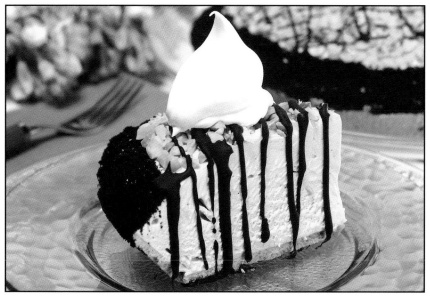

Anutrasized™ Peanut Butter Pie - page 311

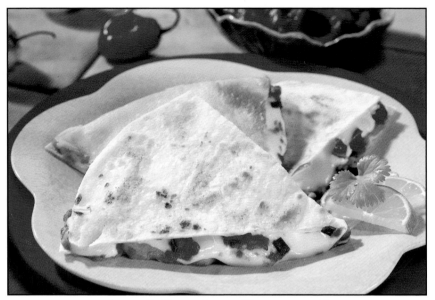

Anutra® Cheesy Quesadillas - page 164

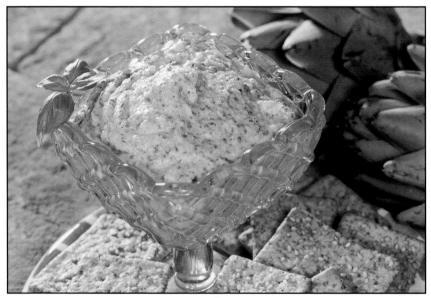

Spinach and Artichoke Anutra® Cream Cheese Dip - page 158

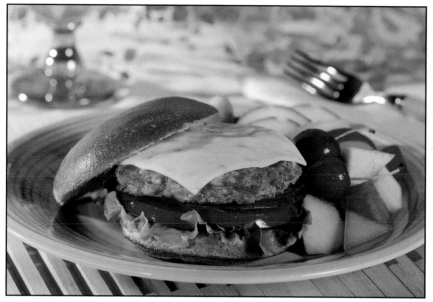

The Anutra® Burger - page 192

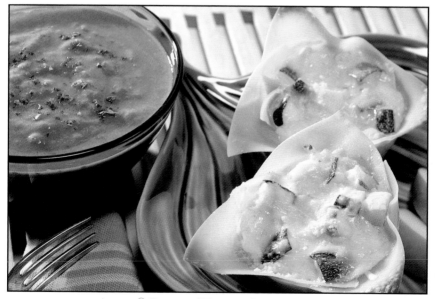

Anutra® Cream of Tomato Soup - page 208
Anutra® Vegetable Quiches - page 150

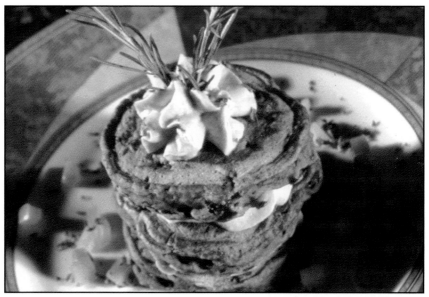

Anutra® Black Bean Pancakes - page 156

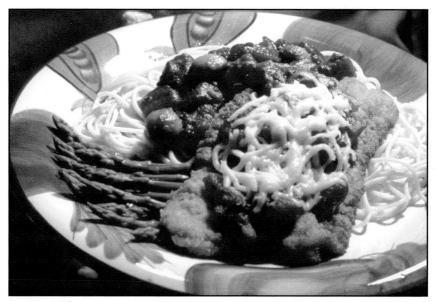

Anutra® Mozzarella & Eggplant Parmesan over Spaghetti with fresh
Asparagus - page 249